Abuse to Abundance

How to Claim Your Mind, Body and Soul

By

Jay Diamond

CONTENTS

Introduction..1

How to Use This Book...1

Ancestral Healing...9

The F Word – Forgiveness...23

Pain is Your Gateway...35

Sex..47

Healing Body Hate...71

Money...83

The Courage to be Intimate.......................................93

Healing my Relationship with Men..........................103

Moving into Abundance...115

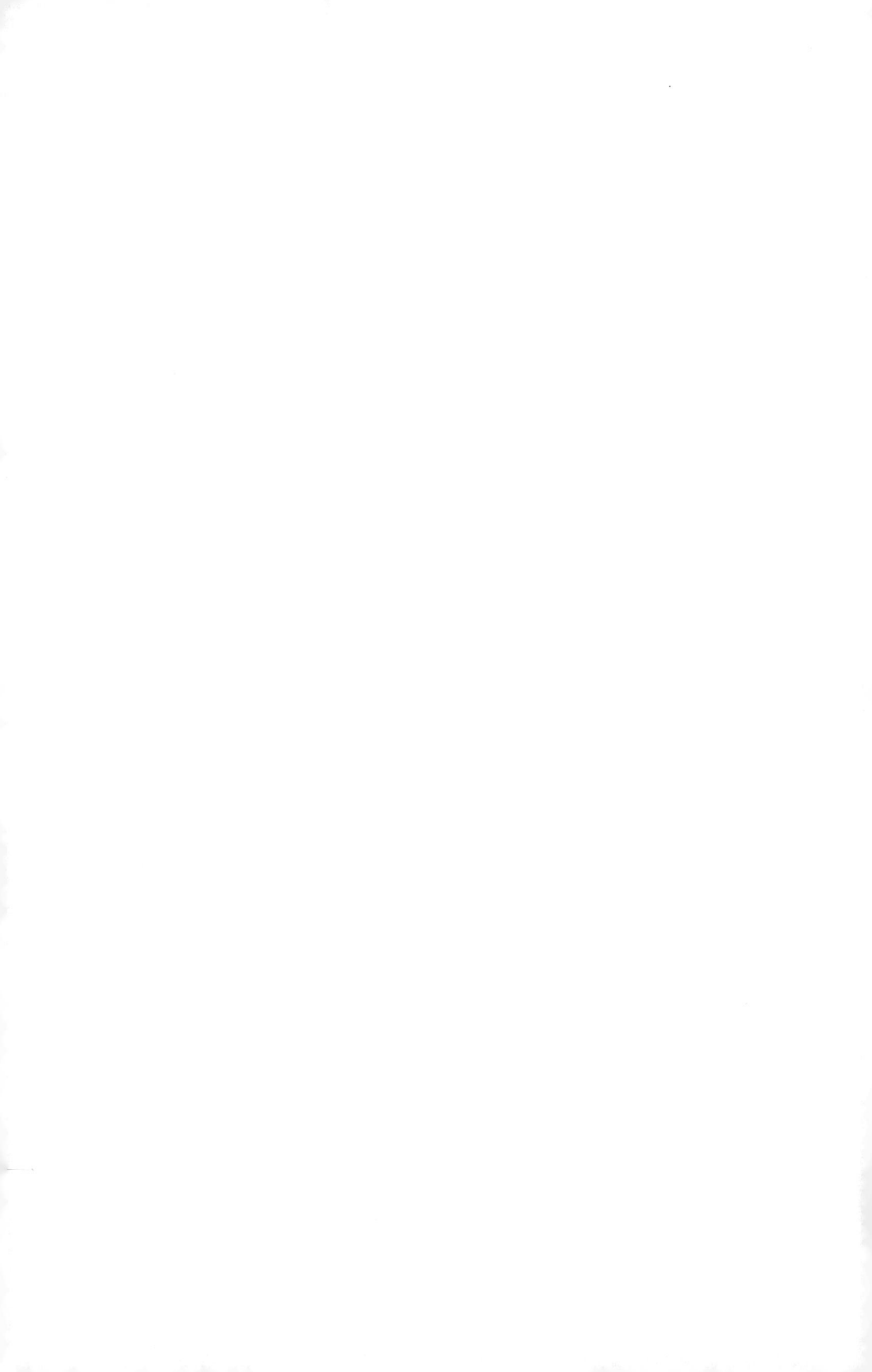

This book is not intended to diagnose, treat, cure, or prevent any disease. This book is not intended as medical advice. This book is provided for informational and educational purposes only, not as a treatment guide or instructions for any diagnosis or condition.

Any diagnosis requires the treatment of a licensed physician. This book is not to be used to substitute for professional medical care. Do not begin any new treatment program without full consent and supervision from a licensed physician. If you have a medical problem, consult a doctor, not this book.

The author offers no guarantee that the ideas in this book are the best therapies for your condition(s). They are simply ideas that the authors felt compelled to write about. Do not rely on this book as final treatment in any condition however mild or severe.

Introduction

How to Use This Book

This is a book for those on a healing journey, overcoming abuse of any kind; emotional, physical, or sexual. The order you read the chapters doesn't matter, you can read from beginning to end or you can start at the chapter that calls to you the most and start there.

I have created a workbook companion for you to use as a journey through this book. Use it to guide you through the healing exercises. It is an invaluable tool that will elevate your healing experience with this book, plus you'll be able to keep all of your new healing tools in one place.

Download it here now:

http://jaydiamond.net/abundanceworkbook/

This book is an instrument to help you grow, from the abuse you experienced to the abundant life you deserve. Abundance is your birth right as a human being, and you do not have to do anything to earn it. You are a sovereign being; you have an innate power in you that cannot be changed by external circumstances. You have the power within you to create the life you desire.

The opportunity to you to shed layers of confusion, pain, and fear to reveal who you truly are underneath is in your hands.

This is your time to heal.

This is your time to transmute pain into power.

This is your time to create your abundant life.

No matter what you have been through, you **can** heal, you **deserve** to heal, and you can **rise** like a phoenix from the ashes.

Claiming Abundance in life is claiming love – self-love, family love, sexual love, health and money as love, security as love, and joy and peace as love.

What I have found in my 20 years as a healer, and about the same amount of time working on my own personal healing, is that there seems to be something about sexual abuse in particular that has far-reaching consequences across a person's life for many years. It does not just affect their sexuality, but also their self-esteem, body image, future relationships, weight, ability to show up in their life purpose, relationship with money, and many other areas.

That said, this book is for all men and women overcoming any kind of abuse.

I have spent years in self-development, working with traditional talk therapies such as Transactional Analysis, counselling, shamanic healing, energy healing, and a whole host of other natural therapies, as well as attending powerful self-development seminars. Each modality was helpful and healing, but I never found anything that would address all the different areas of my healing process in one place.

This book is the place where you will find the different elements of your healing journey all in one place. I could easily write a whole book on each individual technique, but I have broken it down to the essentials, then given you practical steps to move forward in each area.

This book will give you insights into how to move from Abuse to Abundance in various areas of your life, because we deserve to be abundant in *all* ways. I am not afraid to talk about sex, and I'm not afraid to talk about money. I've found with my clients that although these subjects often present huge problems for them, there still seems to be a lot of taboo about tackling these issues head-on. No more; let's rise in love together and claim the abundant life we each deserve.

You are not alone, I will hold your hand throughout this process.

Each chapter will offer you some practical healing techniques that you can do for yourself to help identify what is holding you back, so you can move beyond it. I will also confide in you and share some of my personal stories as a way to assist you on your own healing journey. It'll be like coming to my house for a cup of tea and asking for my advice as a friend and a healer.

I was first told I was psychic in a tarot card reading in my early 20's, and although I meditated with crystals as a teenager and had felt spiritual presence, I didn't really believe it. However, as time moved on, I found myself developing my own healing and psychic abilities, and my clients always had very powerful shifts; quite often life-changing. The more I committed to my own inner healing, the clearer channel I became for healing others. I found myself travelling to sacred places all over the world, connecting with the land and spiritual energies of Hawai'i, the hidden temples of Mexico, the jungles of Peru, the lay lines of Glastonbury, Ashrams and Tantra Masters in India, and so many more. I soaked up spiritual practices across the planet, diving deeper and deeper into the realms of human consciousness. I immersed myself in spiritual teachings.

In my one-to-one healing and workshops, I connect with the spiritual energies of Angels and Ascended Masters, as well as shamanic spirit animals, to help people heal physically, emotionally, and spiritually. Therefore, this book draws on an array of spiritual concepts. I believe we cannot only stay in the realm of the mind to heal the soul; we must also engage the spirit and the heart, and occasionally open up to realms beyond our understanding. I can testify that opening up at this deeper level has given me the most progress in life.

Together we will take a thorough look at your subconscious mind. The subconscious is the part of the mind that holds feelings and beliefs we don't usually have access to. They are present within our minds but are in somewhat of a blind spot. These feelings are our automatic reactions, ancient beliefs long forgotten, and the reason we keep doing something over and over again long after we promised we wouldn't.

The subconscious holds about 90% of our beliefs and feelings, which means we are unaware of 90% of the thoughts and feelings running the show of our lives. We are generally only aware of the top 10% of our thoughts and feelings in the conscious mind!

It is essential to peer into these subconscious thoughts and change them if you are going to succeed in moving from Abuse to an Abundant life. If you only deal with the surface level of thought, you'll get surface-level, short-lived results. We must dive deeper for long-term results.

What you believe at a deep level is what dictates how much money you have, what your relationships are like, what you accept sexually, or why you are still tied to an addiction. This book will help you peel back the layers of your mind, so you can see what you are really dealing with, and then then change it. It is an essential part of your healing process, so when you read the book, do the practical exercises, as these are what will shift you towards an abundant life.

Use the accompanying workbook and apply the bonus exercises given to you. They are all practices I have used with myself and my clients. They will help you; that is what they are for.

DOWNLOAD IT HERE:

http://jaydiamond.net/abundanceworkbook/

I will talk about some of the same concepts from different angles across the book as a way to help you cement these ideas in your mind. After all, repetition is the mother of all skill.

I will also discuss with you healing practices I have personally used to heal at a very deep level. Although we would like to think we can do it all ourselves with a positive mindset, affirmations, and perhaps a couple of counselling sessions, in reality I've found those of us with a more difficult abusive history need more. I think this needs to be said as I come across many people who are not very happy with where they are in life, yet they have never dived deep in to their own healing journey.

If you truly want to move from Abuse to an Abundant life, you will need more than a monthly meditation and occasional yoga class! You can find out more about my in-depth and one to one work at www.jaydiamond.net

I have used many healing modalities, and I personally use Theta Healing™, Vortex Healing™, EFT, Yogic practices, and more with in my workshops and one-to-one sessions. Some of the most significant healing experiences I have had were with plant spirit medicines when I travelled across the globe.

Although some find these plant spirit medicines highly controversial, they have been used by shamans across the world for thousands of years, from Siberia, to the jungles of Brazil, to the cold forests of Europe. These psychedelic plants such as Ayahuasca, Wachuma, and mushrooms are only to be used in a ceremonial fashion with very experienced shamanic healers who know how to navigate the spiritual realms of consciousness.

I am sharing with you some of my stories because they were essential to my own healing; I do not advocate you try this at home by yourself, at all. I travelled all around the world experiencing many different cultures and traditions.

This is the time for us to reclaim our power, and nature has always held gifts and healing for us as humans. In fact, a quarter of all pharmaceutical medicines we use today are derived from plants.

That said, there has been a rise in 'Ayahuasca Tourism' in recent years, and conversations about sustainability, as well as the dangers of simply turning up in a foreign country looking for a cheap 'ceremony' to experience a new high, absolutely need to occur. Although there may be some controversy and we are all still finding our way, it is my belief that Mother Nature is calling us all home to the heart. We must be responsible, mindful, and well-researched in our choices regarding any healing path.

The Western mind is often searching for the 'quick fix,' but this doesn't exist when it comes to long-term healing. Psychedelic plant medicines often go quickly to the shadowed and repressed parts of our being that quietly dictate our lives and make us miserable – shedding light, so these areas can be healed. Some work toward self-development, prior and post this experience, is essential to both prepare the mind and integrate the revelations.

These ancient medicines that grow from the soil must be respected and treated with care, for they open realms of the mind and spirit most of us are unaware of. Despite thousands of testimonials from people who completely overcame depression or addiction, recovered from childhood abuse, and more, some still prefer to demonize these medicines and refer to them as illicit 'drugs.'

Meanwhile there are more than 64,000 deaths a year from prescription drugs in the USA. It is a double standard that doesn't make sense to me, except that pharmaceutical companies profit from prescription drugs.

Due to my own healing practices, I barely ever have the need to take a paracetamol, let alone anything else. I have always preferred a more natural way to heal my pain.

The modern western psychiatric and general medical model is very drug-focused, so drugs are often used to manage the symptoms of mental illness and distress without much attention to finding the underlying cause. Plant medicines such as Ayahuasca seek to identify, express, and release the *underlying cause of distress*, so that it no longer has a strong hold over the consciousness.

To truly move from Abuse to Abundance we cannot simply treat the symptom, we must address the root cause.

Dr. Riba is a world leading professor of pharmacology conducting clinical trials on the effects of Ayahuasca for 20 years. He and his colleagues found that Ayahuasca creates brain activity that helps emotional processing. It can trigger old memories, but it's coupled with increased serotonin (the happy hormone) so that the memory can be processed without being too overwhelming. There are many personal accounts from post-war veterans who say the medicine has eased their PTSD. Other studies found Ayahuasca participants experienced **without recurrence,** the remission of their depression, anxiety disorders, or addictions. Amazingly, they also found it increases the number of *serotonin receptors* in a person.

This discovery means that even if the 'happy hormone,' serotonin, in a person is low, it can be better utilized, as there are more receptors created to switch on the happiness feeling. Those who have used Ayahuasca may feel better, faster, because of this biological shift.

Alternatively, long term use of Prozac-type anti-depressants, actually *decrease* serotonin receptors over time, meaning it gets harder and harder to reach that happy place as the months go by.

With a BSc in psychology, I just love to learn about the scientific findings related to plant spirit medicine; it totally feeds my inner geek. But it's important not to fixate on the science and leave out the **spirit** aspect. These are healing techniques that utilize the spirit realm and the spiritual body for most of their healing. Spiritual gateways are opened, so it's imperative that people don't try to do this without the support of an experienced traditional healer.

I also mention non-psychedelic plant healing such as Bach Flower Remedies and Homeopathy, both of which I have personally found helpful to overcome depression, anxiety (which I dealt with for years), and emotional difficulties. For all types of healing practices, always find qualified and recommended practitioners for healing consultations, although many health food shops now sell home remedies in small amounts.

You must always use your own discernment, trust your gut, and seek recommendations and counsel from those you trust.

This next paragraph is a healing transmission in the tradition of my Theta Healing practice, and you will need to say 'yes' if you would like to receive it. It is at your own free will. We use the word 'command' for certainty.

By reading this paragraph and saying 'yes,' it is commanded that you be sent unconditional love by the creator of all that is to assist you on your healing journey.

Simply say 'yes' now to receive it, and the transmission will be sent to your heart as you read these words. Healing can happen in an instant, and you deserve a miracle in your life.

Will you receive it?

Don't underestimate your own power and intention. Your decision to move from Abuse to Abundance will heal your life.

I send you love and light on your journey. May you be blessed with increase, love, joy, and self-confidence; always.

Jay x

ANCESTRAL HEALING

What secrets and stories does your family carry?

Do you know you carry codes in your blood?

We are all familiar with seeing family members who have the same large nose or open, smiling eyes. It's in their genetic code; that nose - it gets passed down from one generation to the next.

But what about emotions and feelings? We forget about these because we can't see them, yet they're very real, aren't they?

Studies have shown that the grandchildren of holocaust survivors have different stress hormone profiles than their peers, which could make them more likely to have anxiety disorders. Put simply, they were more vulnerable to the effects of stress.

Other studies have shown that if the maternal grandmother was underfed before puberty, her grandchildren were more likely to have diabetes!

How crazy is that? It makes you think, doesn't it?

The experience of your grandparent can influence how *you* feel, and *your* health right now!

Another study on rats showed that when the scent of cherry blossom was paired with an electric shock, the 3rd generation of rats (grandchildren of the original rats) actually **feared the smell of cherry blossom and had more cherry blossom receptors - even if they had never received a shock.**

What does this mean? The new baby rats had a higher awareness for this type of 'danger.' To their grandparents, the smell of cherry blossom meant a bad shock - so the message was sent down the line in the genetic coding to help keep the offspring safe!

Wow!

The 3rd generation rats had a higher stress response **and** had actually changed *genetically* to be more aware of this possible danger.

This is not learned behaviour, it is genetic.

Have you ever had reactions or aversions you can't explain?

Addictions you don't understand?

It could be your genetic coding.

You are the result of hundreds of generations that went before you. They are your ancestors.

There may be coding in your DNA that is supposed to protect you from danger or pain but isn't actually very helpful anymore. This code could show up as an easy trigger for anxiety, an aversion to relationships, or a sabotaging behaviour with money.

I found that many of my clients hold beliefs on an ancestral level that they will be attacked or robbed if they have money, or that they should stay at a low economic level to fit in with their clan (family) or socio-economic class. Humans have a need to belong, so these clients subconsciously reject money to stay safe and remain a part of their clan/ tribe/ family. When we cleared these beliefs, their cash flow increased! Sometimes overnight! Two centuries ago, showing wealth, when your community was poor, could have been a very real threat.

As you move from Abuse to Aoundance, you can ask the questions:

What were my ancestors' beliefs about money?

What were my ancestors' beliefs about marriage?

What were my ancestors' beliefs about health?

Are there any patterns that show up in your family?

Perhaps underachieving (to avoid failure), broken relationships (love = pain), or overeating (to avoid past starvation) that keep showing up in and across your family?

Science is catching up with what shamans, healers, and ancient spiritual traditions have known for centuries: some of the healing you need may actually be connected to your ancestors.

We carry in our bodies the strength, illnesses, tragedies, gifts, understanding, and grief of our ancestors within our genetic coding. Perhaps this information is nature's way of ensuring our survival by preparing us to avoid danger and helping us to develop the particular strengths we need in our environment.

We're usually completely unaware of how these patterns affect us in everyday life, impacting the way we feel about ourselves, our outlook on the world, and the stress we feel. We adopt behaviours that we don't like, but don't know how to stop.

Sometimes we see patterns of addiction, suicide, poor health, anger, low self-esteem, or abuse passed down from generation to generation. From a shamanic perspective, this becomes an energy frequency that is stuck in the energetic body of the person, casting some influence over their thinking or behaviour.

Dealing with this energy frequency is a bit like when a radio is tuned to your favourite station but keeps getting static, messing up your favourite song. The song's still playing, but the static keeps interfering with the clear sound! Your soul's expression is the true song, the pain of your ancestors is the static.

People with traumatic family backgrounds including abuse, neglect, starvation, slavery, and low self-esteem, often benefit from ancestral healing to enhance full and deep personal healing on many levels. The subconscious mind often doesn't know the difference between the message coming from genetics or the message coming from the mind of the person in this lifetime.

We all have genetic programs on human survival that are hundreds or thousands of years old. Some of these are very helpful, such as being alert in the dark in case of danger, staying away from unpredictable animals, and avoiding angry people. We need these programs to keep us safe.

Some programs however are outdated and work against us in modern times; programs like, refusing to let others get close for fear of betrayal, sabotaging money-making schemes for fear of reprisal, or avoiding relationships to prevent chaotic breakups.

In some circles they call healing ancestral patterns 'bloodline work,' and I have found it to be deeply impactful. This is work not just for yourself, but for your children's children. When you embark on this path you are clearing the karma, the actions and reactions of the past, and clearing stuck beliefs and energies in our genetics so that our children can be freer beings.

Free of our burdens, free of our pain, and free of past conditioning. Spiritual and religious traditions all over the world have talked about this freedom for centuries.

By karma, I mean the *impact* of events from the past. This doesn't assign *blame,* but just states that where there's a cause, there is also an effect.

There is something very special about this work I've found, that it not only affects the person receiving the healing, but also creates change within his or her **living** family, promoting more harmony.

Changing myself, on a deep level, has the ability to send out ripples of healing throughout my family. Whether my family knows it or not, I feel and see this to be true. As I change, my world around me changes. As I changed, my family started to shift and change as well.

In a universe where everything is energy, as your beliefs shift internally, what is reflected back to you in your world also shifts. Studies have shown that sending good thoughts to other people can actually affect their autonomic nervous systems. What we think and how we feel affects others!

Most people set about trying to change other people so they can feel better within. The clever person changes their internal world, realizing they can never really control others.

This kind of healing is available to all of us, not just a chosen few.

What ancestral imprints or ancestral issues look like:

- A thread of belief or an issue that affects a number of family members, perhaps all the men, or all the women, or from one generation to the next; for example, not being happy with your body or deep cynicism.

- A problem that won't shift even though you have *proactively worked on yourself first* to heal this issue. Let's not look to our ancestors when we haven't even dealt with our own issues!

- A destructive behaviour that runs across the family, such as incest or addiction. The addiction may show up in different ways for each family member such as gambling, food, drugs, or smoking.

- An illness such as sudden heart disease or breast cancer that happens in the mid-40's.

Many other practitioners and I work with healing ancestral wounds and belief patterns that hold you back from fully enjoying your life. This work has great results. I found that psychoactive plant medicines, Theta Healing, and Vortex Healing can create deep and quick transformational changes to dissolve old programming.

When this trapped ancestral energy is freed up, many experience a discovery of gifts that lay dormant in the ancestral heritage, or deep within them. This realization could come in the form of revitalized energy, increased personal power, the flowering of musical and psychic abilities, or a sudden affiliation with a country, culture, or dance.

Feeling safe

Many religious and spiritual traditions all over the world, including Celtic, Mayan, Ancient Greek, and African tribal groups have rituals and ceremonies to honour their ancestors and attract guidance, good luck, and blessings.

The ancestral rituals are usually done through prayer, mediation, creation of art, music, food and ceremony, or a special day such as the Catholic All-Saints Day.

However, when I first heard about calling my ancestors into a healing ritual I would **not** do it.

"No way am I bringing those crazy b*stards into my healing," I exclaimed. "Why would I want to bring dysfunctional, dead people into my life! I've got enough that are living!"

Clearly, I didn't quite understand the deal. Firstly, calling in and connecting with the energy of your ancestors is not an invitation to bring any old ghost into your home!

Discernment is important and needed. I always call on "my highest light and love ancestors." Just because someone passes over, it doesn't automatically make them a saint. They can be just as cantankerous dead as well as alive!

On passing, many souls go through a process of evaluation, and may choose spiritual evolution, healing, and understanding from that point. However, others may decide not to and stay stuck as the personality they had in human form for a while longer, according to many mediums.

If I call the ancestors of highest light and love vibration, I can't go wrong, and I won't attract a random aunty with a bad attitude.

For me, ancestral ritual and healing is calling in spiritual guidance and support from beings in my bloodline that know what it is like to incarnate in human form, and all the ups and downs we have on this Earth plane. I don't experience any sort of apparition or ghost visit; usually it's just a gentle feeling of presence, or I just know that I have asked them to be there with me in my prayer or healing session. My ancestors have an earthly understanding of my family relationships, problems, and patterns, so they can be good advisors and helpers.

It was explained to me that I did not have to call in my Grandparents who were neglectful or abusive to me in my present life; but that I could call on the greater ancestral line to help me heal the wounds of these relationships in my present life. It was nice to think that there was family somewhere that cared, and cared enough to help, even if they were dead and I was quite dubious at first!

The unfolding of female grief

I felt the warmth of white light wash over my body, as I rested into a gentle relaxation. The Ayahuasca settled gently in my body and I felt light and floaty.

A twinge in my stomach became more and more uncomfortable, until I writhed around on the floor clutching my belly, like I had food poisoning.

This plant spirit intelligence worked through my body, drawing out negative energy trapped in the cells of my body, bringing it to the stomach so that it could be expelled either by vomiting or diarrhoea. It's a very clever system that can take minutes or hours, but it's often pretty uncomfortable.

Without warning, my focus shifted as I realised something huge was about to happen. What I refer to and experience as 'me,' Jay Diamond, disintegrated and unravelled.

My body and mind peeled back in layers, over and over again. I felt myself shaved open like a continuous unfolding of lotus petals. A never-ending blooming of a flower, my body prised open from the core, then folding ever outwards.

From this core; boundless sorrow erupted like a tidal wave. I felt the grief and anguish of women of all ages, uncontrollably expressed through me. I shapeshifted, feeling myself as a grandmother, aged, worn, and experienced; then as a child, small, light, and open. I felt myself as a middle-aged woman, grounded and wise; then as a teenage girl, growing and curious. They released their grief through me, as me.

I wailed with the grief of a mother holding her dead new-born baby in her arms. My heart shattered with the horror of the grandmother witnessing the murder of her family.

Like a repeated punch to the stomach, blow after blow, I was desolate and panicked; I was helpless and guilt-stricken; I was terrified beyond repair.

It was the most intimate and private of human pain; laid open without a hiding place.

I could feel the broken women who never recovered, the women of my bloodline who never got to process their grief. The plant spirit helped me to cross a portal of time and space, turning the key and unlocking the door of the deepest wounds of my female ancestors. Timelines merged, lifetimes blurred, and I freed myself, by freeing them. An entire lineage of healing took place.

Spiritually shedding the stories, the pain, and the programming of the ancient past, I released the ancestral pattern of feminine grief in my body. I rested my weary bones as I put my hand on my heart with gratitude for the healing.

I had no idea this kind of healing was even possible. I felt called to psychoactive plant medicines because although I had progressed so far in my life, I still felt stuck. Life had thrown me a curve ball, and I didn't know how to recover. My family relationships were a mess, my confidence was low, and issues I thought I had resolved resurfaced.

I felt both strongly called and deeply nervous, so I did research over a number of months before I decided to take the plunge. It's not a path for the faint-hearted.

There are many ways we can connect with our ancestors, though deep healing often requires more focused attention with a practitioner.

This particular healing was extreme. It cleared many generations of ancestral pain compressed into 30 minutes. But, I would rather have a hard half-hour than years of feeling quietly dissatisfied.

Certainly not all ancestral healing looks or feels like this particular session, so don't worry. Some ancestral healing merely feels like a weight has been lifted off your shoulders, or finally gaining perspective on a reoccurring issue in your life. However you decide to do it, dealing with ancestral wounds brings great rewards and peace into your everyday life.

The mother wound, the father wound, and ancestral healing

Two key themes you can focus on in your healing journey with your ancestral line are the Mother Wound and the Father Wound.

Our relationship with our parents, whether they were present in childhood or not, is foundational to our experience of ourselves and our experience of life. It impacts our belief system and well-being well into adulthood.

The mother wound and father wound are phrases that relate to the limiting beliefs or learned behaviours that are unhelpful due to our relationship, or lack thereof, with our parents. This includes beliefs such as, 'I will never be enough,' 'I am not lovable,' or 'I must assert my authority.'

The way our parents behaved is usually reflective of how their parents behaved towards them.

Is there a pattern of physical or emotional abuse in your father line, through your father, grandfather, or great-grandfather? Or perhaps a pattern of emotional withdrawal in your mother line, by way of your mother, grandmother, or great-grandmother?

Get curious. Your experience of your great-grandmother in her 80's might be very different than your mother's experience of her as a child.

In a patriarchal society, a woman may have learned to survive by minimizing her power, being manipulative, or keeping secrets as a way to protect herself in a society that didn't allow her to be in her full power. This, of course, affects her relationships with others. Conversely, living in a patriarchal society might cause a woman to become angry, distant, and withdrawn.

Men may have learned to survive by being aggressive, domineering, or dismissive in order to maintain power and, possibly, to hide the fear and the weight of always having to be strong to survive. Conversely, they may become compliant, malleable, or withdrawn as a way to get by hassle-free.

Families that survived war, often did so without any kind of therapeutic process to help them integrate their overwhelming grief, fear, or anger. And many of our grandparents survived world wars!

So where does this energy and emotion go?

Down the bloodline of course.

What it means to be a man, or what it means to be a woman -- the roles we play because of our gender - are largely learned behaviours.

We learn not just by the society around us, but by our parents. Being a man in one family might mean being a provider, encouraging your children, and uplifting your wife. In another, it might mean paying no attention to others' needs, being emotionally absent, and drinking after a hard day. If you don't address the wounds that travel down your family line, it is difficult to become the man or woman that you are not only capable of being, but who you truly are without the roles that were passed down to you.

As children, we are like sponges, taking in everything going on around us and learning how to be a human. Our environment becomes a blueprint for life, whether we like the blueprint or not. Your childhood experiences were not your choice, but how you choose to live your life now is your responsibility.

Identify the patterns in your mother line and father line so you can heal them. You do not need to repeat their patterns. It is now time for you to be free of it.

As you heal the feminine energies, this will increase your ability to receive goodness from life and be supported, by people, by finances, by life. This is because the feminine energy is receptive.

As you heal the masculine energies you can balance action and rest, improve your ability to manifest your desires, and feel comfortable with success. The masculine energy is active.

You'll find practices to look at these patterns at the end of this chapter.

This type of healing helps you move from Abuse to Abundance as you become free of what has held you back on a family level.

The truth is, we are always doing our best at the level of understanding we have. When you know better, you do better. If your parent had the skills, the self-love, and the confidence to do better for you, they would.

But perhaps they didn't. They did what they knew how to do, whether that was being a fantastic, loving role model, or a heroin-addicted, neglectful parent who never said they loved you. It's a hard pill to swallow, but you can't change the past, and you can't change anyone else.

When you accept this and stop trying to make the past different, you will feel a weight lift off your shoulders, and have more energy to give to yourself.

You may never get the recognition or the apology you deserve, but as long as you keep needing this affirmation from another person you will never be free.

Freedom comes when you give yourself what you needed as a child; when you recognize and accept yourself for all you are and all you have overcome.

Make a decision to love yourself and make your own journey from Abuse to Abundance, right now.

Your life will change.

Because YOU are born and destined for greatness.

That's why you're reading this. That's why you were called to this book. It has nothing to do with me and everything to do with you.

If you found yourself in the pages of this book, I'm willing to bet you made something great of yourself. You might not be where you want to be, but you sure don't look like where you've come from!

You are here because now you're willing to evolve, and you need to honour yourself for how far you have come!

But here's the thing, you may not have stepped into your total potential because of the shadows of your family pain and old beliefs still hang over you.

Abuse

My grandmother loved me. She chain-smoked an[d]... shake. The child of strong Catholic Irish immigrants, as... affair with a school teacher, and they eventually married.

I'm sure this relationship was frowned upon at first, but... way with money that won people to his side, even her parents. She had no idea of the life she would go on to live, or that this man, so many years older than her, was a paedophile.

My grandmother loved me, but she didn't know how to protect me. Her will was broken long before I came along, and she tried so hard to make me happy. As a child, all I knew how to do was love, and I saw no fault in her, but through my ancestral healing work, I discovered that silently, quietly, in the back of my mind, I *had* seen her pain.

And even though I didn't realise it, as a little girl, I swore to myself I would never be trapped in a relationship like she was. And so, I was single for a very long time trying to avoid the pain she had.

Exercise:

With your journal:

What events or behaviours have you seen in your family that make you say, "I never want to end up like that!"

What unhealthy patterns can you detect across your family? Perhaps there's a tendency to keep secrets, get angry easily or unhappy marriages.

Which beliefs or new behaviours could you adopt to avoid this kind of pain continuing inside your life?

Write out what you are choosing now:

E.g. If you see a pattern of avoiding communication and back stabbing you may choose a new belief:

I choose to have clear and honest communication in my life.

If many family members are addicted to gambling, alcohol or overwork, you may choose the new belief:

I choose to live free of addiction.

What do you need to do, be, have, find, and align yourself with to make this your new truth?

Do you need a support group, a therapist, to learn all you can about communication skills, or work life balance? Don't just write a new belief, take action on it to make the change real.

You will start to understand why some things have been so hard for you to get over, and know to improve your relationships, self-esteem, or finances.

Summary:

- Studies have shown that the experience of our grandparents could affect our physical and emotional health.

- Ancestral healing may hold the key to feeling free when you've tried everything else.

- Assessing your mother line and father line can inform you about how you show up in your role as a man or a woman, revealing what you may like to change.

THE F WORD – FORGIVENESS

"Fear binds the world. Forgiveness sets it free." - Lesson 332 - A Course in Miracles.

Refusing to forgive is refusing to heal.

I know that's a strong a statement, but as you continue your healing journey, you will find it to be true. Every spiritual tradition teaches forgiveness because it is a necessary pre-requisite to your freedom.

The ego likes to think, "If I forgive someone it means they win and I lose," as if the person who holds out the longest has the most power. Or alternatively, "What they did was wrong, forgiving is like saying it was ok!"

When we withhold forgiveness, the person we are upset with can take up space in our head, rent-free. A part of our energy is still connected to them, and a simple thought of them can spark anger or sorrow.

Forgiveness is not letting someone off the hook, nor saying that their actions didn't hurt you. It is not a free pass for others to walk all over you without apology, or a way for you to not take responsibility for your own boundaries. Forgiveness is not simply saying the words 'I forgive you,' but still secretly harbouring resentment. And it is definitely not pretending all is well and rebuilding relationships with dysfunctional people.

True forgiveness is accepting and understanding that humans are imperfect, and that this is part of life. It is deciding to let them go because **you** want be free, because **you** no longer wish to carry anger, hurt, and resentment within you. It is taking care of your own heart. Forgiveness is allowing the pain you feel to return to love, which is your true nature.

Forgiveness is an act of loving yourself enough to move on to an abundant future, regardless of what happened in the past.

Love is your true nature, and when love is blocked, you will not feel at peace.

Unfortunately, simply saying, "I forgive them," doesn't mean true forgiveness. You have truly forgiven someone when the emotional charge has gone when they come to your mind. This is why when you truly forgive someone, the intrusive thoughts about them, the memories and the emotions start to fade away. You have severed the emotional attachment to them and replaced it with love for yourself.

Forgiving someone who abused you takes strength, courage, and time, especially when you've spent twenty or so years believing you could not and should not forgive. It can feel like an impossible task, and you probably think, "Why should I!? They don't deserve to be forgiven!"

But the thing is, when you still hold anger for someone because they don't deserve to be forgiven, it's like drinking poison and waiting for the other person to die.

You are the one holding the anger, you are the one feeling the pain, not them. Reliving old pain over and over will not make them say, 'sorry,' and it won't make them see the error of their ways either. Your pain won't change the past.

But if you don't let go of the pain, it will change you.

Don't drink someone else's poison and expect them to die, because they won't. They will still be out there trying to make the best of their lives, while you hold yourself back. Even if you think you are making them pay for what they did, you are **still** the one drinking the poison. It doesn't make sense to withhold peace from yourself any longer.

Forgiveness - the F word - is your route to freedom.

When you've carried pain for a long time, you can come up with a lot of reasons about why you can't forgive:

It might feel like:

What they did was ok. It's not, so I can't forgive them.

I feel like I'm letting other people down who this has happened to if I forgive.

I deserve to feel bad, it was my fault really.

What will people say if I forgive something so awful?

If I forgive, people will think I lied.

I want to make them pay.

If I forgive, I will have to move on, and I'm not sure what to do with myself.

If I forgive, I will have to claim my own power, and that feels scary.

I've built my life on this story; who am I without this?

I need anger to fuel me.

Forgiving is passive. I will get abused again if I forgive.

And so on.

As a child, we feel disempowered when we are under someone else's control or authority, or when our caregivers withhold love and security. When a child is physically, emotionally, or sexually abused, this leads to a feeling of disempowerment. This leads on to anger, because that's the way the mind knows to reassert itself and feel powerful again.

Even if at the time we didn't feel anger, this sense of being disempowered or not getting our needs met will **lead** to anger. Sometimes we don't even know the anger is there because we have repressed it; the whole situation is just too horrible to think about, so we pack it all away, anger and all.

However, the energy of anger has a job, and it's job is to attack! It doesn't care who or why. Anger will turn on others, or it will turn on you. This is how illness starts, or depression, or panic attacks. Hate and anger are poisons that don't belong in your body.

When we hold on to deep anger, people tend to avoid us and we don't know why. It's because the anger seeps through, unknown to us, but others can *feel* it. You may be easily triggered to anger or depression because of suppressed anger, and not even know why this is happening.

The anger will keep doing its job of attacking until you address its cause -- the feeling of disempowerment.

Can you see why forgiveness is essential in order to move from Abuse to Abundance?

Although you can't change what someone else did, you can change what you choose to believe about yourself and change your life because of it. You don't have to live like you did in the past; you can create your own life from now on.

Who do you need to forgive so you can move on? It all starts and ends with you.

The change you seek is within you

"Everything in the Universe is within you. Ask all from yourself." - Rumi, Sufi philosopher.

"The kingdom of God lies within." - Luke 17:21, The Holy Bible.

"All light and all darkness exist within us" - San Pedro, (transmission to me.)

The idea that the change you seek, and the life you experience starts within you, is a philosophy taught in spiritual traditions all across the world. But what does this notion really mean?

We are spiritual beings having a human experience, rather than human beings having a spiritual experience.

Each of us has a soul. When you ask the question, "Who am I?" you may come up with all kinds of answers. You might mention your name, job, or family role - son, brother, sister, or mother. Qualities such as being a good friend, open-hearted, anxious, or confident might be your focus. How about where you're from, your social status, your hobbies, or how much you earn?

These are the things we typically reply with when we ask, "Who am I?" But what if we took those things away from you? If you change your name, are you still you?

If you change jobs, move cities, your sibling dies, or you are no longer as confident as you were - are you still you?

Yes, of course you are.

Because who you are really is none of the labels or roles you play in your life. There is something in you that is eternal and is beyond **all** of those things.

That something is your soul.

Your soul is a spark of Universal Consciousness; I call that consciousness God. You are a spark of God. Universal Consciousness is all there is; it is a vast field of infinite intelligence that runs through everything in the cosmos. It holds all the feelings, all the emotions, all the possibilities, experiences, the past, the present, and the future. It is the energy of life, and the places between lives.

Like the radio waves that make your phone work, you can't see this force, but it's there, and every religion and spiritual philosophy has been trying to help us understand this for thousands of years, so there must be *something* to it!

But why is this concept important to understand?

Because if we are a droplet of water in the ocean of Universal Consciousness, then we have access to this Universal Consciousness. It is within us and it's what we are made up of.

There is a place inside you where you have access to everything in the universe! Essentially all of life exists with us. Like a hologram, you can access all the information and pictures from just one fragment, the good the bad, and the ugly. This is what the ancient yogis knew, and how they mapped out our solar system long before telescopes were discovered.

When we go within to heal the place that feels rejected, or unlovable, or insignificant, our whole life changes. When we go within, it's like upgrading the hard drive of the computer instead of just pressing the same buttons expecting things to change.

How many times have you pressed the same old buttons to make something work instead of upgrading the hard drive or making the change within you? How many times have you changed external relationships but you still acted the same old way? You said you would stop drinking, but really just switched to beer instead of spirits? Or made new money, only to spend it all within a week?

When I'm with clients, we focus on healing the root issue of what's keeping them stuck. Because you are connected to all that is, when you change by going within, everything around you changes. This is how miracles happen, relationships are saved, and illnesses dissipate.

Change your beliefs, change your life. Heal your heart, heal your life.

Instead of reaching 'out there' to forgive, reach in. Forgive; forgive it all. And forgive again. Can you love and accept all the difficult emotions inside of you?

Love is a healing balm to be offered to yourself. Love the place that hurts; offer love and comfort to the anger, the sadness, or humiliation instead of rejecting it and pushing it away. The feeling is calling out to be loved and accepted by you. When you love these seemingly unlovable places, you will heal.

It took a long time for me to fully forgive the grandfather who abused me. It happened in stages and layers, and I never imagined the depths of my soul I would have to go to in order to do it.

The layers of letting go

An ant peacefully stomped by, making his way across the grass. The blue sky opened gloriously above me, but here I was again, gripping my stomach stuck in nausea and not able to puke. Stroking my belly, with head flopped to one side, "Come on, come on, now, come up," I coaxed. The Wachuma, a South American plant spirit medicine, made me feel ill, and I felt grumpy.

Something was stuck.

"Do you need help?" enquired one of our gentle shamanic healers with a tender smile. She lovingly guided me to look into this feeling of sickness and communicate with it. To ask, "What was going on?"

This is a wonderful technique to use with any symptom. Get quiet and ask your body, "What is happening here? What do you need?" You will be surprised at how clear the answers are.

Silenced by shock, I was suddenly face-to-face with the man who abused me as a child.

Although he'd been dead for over ten years, I could feel his spirit as though he stood right in front me.

To my disappointment, despite all the healing, hours of therapy, and consciously working on forgiving this man for what he did, the plant spirit medicine showed me there was still an energetic link connecting me to him. A part of me still hadn't let go.

I honestly believed until that point that I had fully forgiven him and was free. His presence completely freaked me out!

"All light, and all dark exists within us," said the medicine. "Go within."

"He was looking for love," was the message I received.

It dawned on me that this broken, dysfunctional man did hideous things because he was so devoid of love inside of himself. Those who are truly full of love cannot hurt another.

It is the lack of love that causes what we call darkness and dysfunction.

This is one of the reasons why I love and respect our beloved teacher plants. The Wachuma spirit bridged me into the Universal Consciousness. In that moment, I could see the man who hurt me, not from my wounded heart, but from the elevated perspective of the Divine. When I saw and felt this situation through the eyes of love, I took no offence because I finally and deeply got it, that hurt people hurt people, and that is not my fault.

I was reconnected to love.

Instead of hating him, droplets of compassion fell from my eyes. How separated from love he must have been to act in such a way.

"The wound is where the light gets in." - Rumi

Long ago, I had given my power away to that man, and I clawed it back in pieces. Now I was ready to let more love flow inside of me than ever before. I didn't hate him. I didn't hate my past. I just accepted it.

I ordered any energetic links from me to him to be released and dissolved. I called all of my power back to me - physically, emotionally, and spiritually. Then I took a log to the open fire and asked the fire spirit to burn, burn, burn anything in me still tied to this situation and this man, and finally release me, once and for all.

As the log hit the flames, a rush of life-force ripped through my body like a tidal wave, and I dropped to my knees sobbing, "It's gone, it's gone." I felt like I was breathing for the first time.

Here's the thing; rather than being a straight line from A to B, moving from Abuse to Abundance is a healing journey that operates like a spiral. We move down into deeper layers of healing at the rate our mind is ready to let go of the behaviours, beliefs, and trapped feelings that no longer serve us.

At the first layer we may decide that we want to change how we feel and no longer carry the past with us, at the second we may approach forgiveness, at the third we may release resentment, at the fourth we may accept and embrace what is, and at the fifth level unveil the compassion in our heart; and so on.

As we heal, we reach a new level of awareness and understanding about ourselves and about the nature of life itself. We learn deeper and deeper lessons that we cannot comprehend the first time around.

Don't be disheartened if your journey takes time, or you revisit old patterns and beliefs that you thought you had cleared. This is all part of the process, and it's worth every minute of your time.

When you have forgiven, your relationships will deepen, your self-sabotaging behaviours will start to fall away, and you will feel the universal stream of love in your heart once again.

Let go, and start afresh.

to help you forgive:

Thank you, God/ Creator/ Universe,

For bringing me to this point on my journey to learn about forgiveness. Great spirit, I know how forgiveness will free me, heal me, and release me.

I ask that you come into my heart right now. And each and every day, teach me how to forgive _____ (say the person's name or the situation). I am willing even when I don't know how.

I am in pain, and I don't want to carry it any longer, lift this burden from me, Great Spirit. Show me the error in my thinking; remove the fear and anger and hurt in my heart; show me how to forgive, for I cannot do it alone.

I need you, I welcome you, and I ask you to be here with me now and surround me with your love. Cover me in your strength, let me feel your holy support.

Thank you for coming into my heart and letting me feel your love for me like a warm glow. Let me be strengthened by you. Show me how to feel safe enough to let go.

Thank you for showing me how it feels to completely forgive _____ (say the person's name or the situation) and live out the rest of my days in total freedom. Show me how to move on.

Thank you for showing me how to feel I am worthy of forgiveness, and that I can remove the grief of holding on to pain for so long. Thank you that I now see this situation through your eyes, Great Spirit. Thank you for this healing; for transforming me, healing me, and loving me.

Thank you, thank you, and thank you. It is done.

Repeat this prayer as often as wanted or needed.

Summary:

- When you won't forgive you are drinking the poison and expecting the other person to die.

- Your soul is eternal and you have access to all the unconditional love in the universe.

- Healing is a spiral, we revisit old lessons at deeper levels.

PAIN IS YOUR GATEWAY

Many people live a mediocre life. They don't question the beliefs and assumptions that have been handed down to them by their family or community, television, or newspapers. We are generally caught up in the path we are told we should have: that we need to go to school, get a job, get a car, get a partner, have a family, get a promotion, get a better car, go on a holiday, work hard until you retire, slow down, read the paper, and die.

Naturally people crave security and comfort, and they will often choose to stay in a mediocre or unhappy relationship or job rather than take a risk and live the life they really want. Their natural talents and passions are suppressed because they aren't seen as important and may interfere with the path they were told to take.

Does any of this sound familiar?

Because in the West, we don't like to talk about death, we hide from the fact that we have limited time. We just go on and on, following what we've been told will make us happy, as if our days aren't numbered, whether or not we are actually happy.

We keep up the pretence and try to fit in as best as we can, shrugging our shoulders and saying, "Well, that's life!"

Pain will shatter all of this.

As I stood by the edge of the road in Brixton, my legs began to give way under me. Leaning on the wall for support, I tried to make sense of the phone call. My brother had experienced some sort of heavy psychotic episode, terrified my mother, and tried to extort money. Things were said that shattered our family as we knew it.

My world turned in a minute. I just shook.

We had tried to get him help for a long time, to no avail. Over the years, he had become increasingly incoherent; he neglected himself and was erratic. It was impossible to get through to him or talk sense into him.

Unless you've lived through dealing with a family member with complex mental health needs, it's hard to understand what a messy, emotionally burning process it can be.

Over the next months I tried to coordinate his social workers and mental health support with little progress, whilst also trying to deal with the psychological mess of accusations, delusions, shock, and fear. It was hard to know where truth ended and lies began. Everything was a mess. I was a mess.

During this time, I slept with my phone at my side, terrified I would get a call to tell me he was dead, had been beaten up because he was erratic, or had hurt someone. My skin was sensitive and my breathing was erratic; in fact, my whole body was on red alert. I worried obsessively, and when I closed my eyes all I could see in the movie of my mind was his body being lowered into the ground.

Every time the phone rang, I was gripped with terror, convinced something had happened to him.

It got so bad that at night, I would cry myself to sleep in fear and grief. I felt confused about what was happening, and exhausted with trying to find a solution. My breathing became slow and shallow as I eventually slept, with the feeling of no longer wanting to live in a world with so much darkness.

About a year before, I had moved to London with dreams of becoming a radio presenter and DJ. I set up my life pretty well. I worked out at the gym to deal with my anxiety after my boyfriend left; I looked good, and I felt like I had my shit together. I was networking, playing on a great radio station, and DJing in some pretty cool clubs. I was really finding my way to success.

But I didn't cope well when this episode happened. Things were said and done that caused me to question life as I had known it, and I was worried that none of us were coping well with the aftermath.

The situation brought up every unhealed wound that I thought I had put to rest. I thought I'd dealt with most of my issues relating to sexual abuse, my confidence, and my relationships with my parents. Turns out, I was wrong.

Life pulled the rug out from under my feet, and I was left wondering how to deal with a barrage of old memories, emotions, fears, and resentments.

I was faced with a choice: go deeper into wounds I didn't know I had and face the heartbreak, fear, and relentless ocean of grief, or stuff it all back down.

My confidence plummeted, and my mind was so foggy from all of the stress, that I actually couldn't remember information properly or juggle the different areas of my life like I had before. I started making mistakes and getting overwhelmed easily. I couldn't focus on work or anything else. The problem was, I looked exactly the same on the outside, but on the inside, I was a hot mess.

It was hard to explain to people how bad it was without a long family history lesson or revealing some dark secrets I didn't want to share. So, I said the minimum and bit my lip so I wouldn't cry. I put on the mask of 'I'm ok,' when I was far from it.

Because of the strain on us all, family relationships fell apart and I felt increasingly isolated. But as the months went by, I did my best to live life while being quietly broken inside. I wanted to be strong; I hated feeling broken.

A New York summer

I have always had strong intuitive impulses when it comes to travel, and I felt a powerful pull to go back to New York. Each time I have felt this gut instinct in my life and followed it, good things have happened.

I reconnected with old music contacts and DJed at parties. I tried to meditate and go to yoga classes to fight the anxiety and profound sadness in my heart. I was desperate to feel normal again and make sense of life somehow, so I kept myself busy.

I expected weeks of sun, but I soon discovered that summers in New York are full of thunder and rain.

On the 4th floor of a small apartment in Brooklyn, I could smell the dampness of a storm brewing. The windows were wide, telling tales on the broken air conditioning, and the sky was thick with grey. It was a quiet day; no one around, and nothing to do to keep me busy.

Do you know how it feels to have a busy life and feel utterly alone?

I sat in a corner and wept, asking God to please help me, to take the pain away in my heavy heart, and show me what to do. I cried, begged, and pleaded until I could find no more words to say. I was completely broken.

Open.

Gulping down grief through humid air, I was completely broken open like water through a dam. There was a deep crack in my soul I couldn't hide anymore, and no matter how hard I tried to hold it together I just wasn't strong enough to hold it.

But, they say, the crack is where the light gets in. In life, this crack is often disguised as sheer desperation; waking up in your own vomit after another drinking spree, a spell in jail, or finding out your illness is serious.

The hard truth is, the house that was my life was built on sand. I had made a good life for myself - good job, great friends, gym membership, and a few fun DJ gigs - but I still had beliefs and behaviours that sabotaged my relationships, success, and self-respect. My foundations were not solid, and I needed to be upgraded if I were to be truly happy.

My heart had to be opened if I was to fulfil my potential.

Why pain is your gateway

The pain that could have broken me was my opportunity to grow into the greatest version of myself I was yet to become.

What I know now for sure is life had a plan for me, and life has a plan for you. At the time, I felt like I was being punished, or that a stress-free, fun life is something that happens for other people, but would never happen for me.

In the middle of your mess, it's hard to believe that God truly cares, but what I learned is that everything in your life is calling you to the highest version of yourself, even if you don't understand it yet.

Life is always trying to bring you to higher ground.

On that stormy, hot day, I genuinely cried out to God from the bottom of my heart. I didn't know it at the time, but it was a turning point for me.

Many people report that when they look back, their most difficult experience was a turning point in their lives for the better. A sincere call for help with no ego, but rather pure surrender to allow whatever needs to happen, to occur, to create change.

Letting go of control and surrendering to a higher power, essentially saying, "I'm too exhausted, I'm too hurt, I don't know what to do, and I can't do it anymore. *Please show me!*" never goes unheard.

When you give up your control, the belief that your life or other people should be the way you think they should, when you let go of asking why and instead ask life to show you the way, a new grace and guidance pours over your life.

If you can let the pain transform you, instead of reduce you, it will be your gateway. Accept it, breathe into it, don't reject it, then let it pass and you can be healed.

Gently, I went deeper into spiritual practices, and listened all the time to Joel Osteen, Joyce Meyer, TD Jakes, and Abraham Hicks and filled my heart with positive words and concepts.

It's funny because I had always been afraid of the 'J word.' I was happy to call on the Indian deity Ganesh - the aspect of God that removes obstacles; or meditate to connect to 'the creator,' but would literally squirm in my seat or bolt the room if someone said, "Jesus."

There has been such misuse of the J word - with war, fear mongering, judgement, and pain inflicted by humans - all in the name of Jesus, that churchy stuff scared the 'bejesus' out of me. My experience as a kid in church was that it bored me to tears; and anyway, I just didn't believe in a God that wanted people to go to hell, or a Jesus that supported that.

But during this time, I began to develop my own relationship with Yeshua. (That's Jesus' name in Hebrew, and I like it a lot!) by watching videos on YouTube! I kept watching these teachers because something I couldn't explain was giving me the peace I desperately needed, even if in 30-minute YouTube video bursts. Over the next few years, my connection with him grew and grew. He, Mother Mary, and Mary Magdalene would often show up in my healing work with clients.

Within a year, I was guided to plant spirit medicines. I had asked for healing, and the path began to open. I travelled to different parts of the world, exploring the consciousness of my mind, and healing my broken heart in the deepest way I'd ever known.

I quickly learned that my heartbreak was much more than my present personal hurting. I discovered experientially that past lives and genetic family patterns can plague a person for generations also.

I left my radio work because it wasn't feeding my soul anymore. After years of keeping my healing practice as a hobby, I stepped up into this role with confidence. I accepted that I am here to change lives.

I realised my pain was meant to transform me. My experiences have made me more compassionate and comfortable, calling others into their highest potential. If I can heal, you can too.

Whether I liked it or not, I was set on a better trajectory for my life by being broken open.

I got the chance to assess: Where am I now? Who am I now? Where do I want to be in my life? Am I on track? What isn't working in my life? And most importantly, what do I need to do to change it?

By being isolated from family I was freed from my usual roles and routines with others, and free of their expectations and mine.

I got to recreate myself and build my life from the ground up, so I could be truly happy. Life hadn't given me firm foundations, so I developed my tools box and made my own. My way.

There are gifts for you on the other side of hard times.
Pain is your gateway.

But to get free, you have to tell the truth. If you're going to lie to yourself that you have nothing to do with the partners you keep picking, that getting trashed every weekend isn't really a problem, or your anger is because other people are just stupid, you're blocking your own healing.

If you don't allow yourself to tell the truth on how you really feel - be it out of control, lonely, or weak - how can you ever get the support you deserve? Admitting these things feels tough because it is like death to the ego!

The ego is all the beliefs about who you think you are, and the identity you have constructed for yourself. Your ego needs you to keep on the false mask of 'I'm ok,' because its only job is to keep you safe in any way it sees fit. Quite frankly, it doesn't give a sh*t if you are happy.

To the ego, showing weakness is death, because that's what happened to our ancestors if they showed fear when they were hunting wild animals to eat. The mammalian part of your brain, the part that deals with quick reactions when you feel any kind of threat, doesn't know times have changed now. So, you get stuck in a loop: Show no fear! Show no weakness, or I'll get eaten!

But, we have to learn to tell the truth despite the fear if we want to create an abundant, happy life.

For people who have been sexually, physically, or emotionally abused, naming your emotions can be very difficult because you had to suppress them in the past, and maybe even in the present in order to not fall apart.

You may have numbed yourself in response to the abuse, or the feelings about yourself, or the feelings about life after abuse.

Learning to name emotions other than the standard anger, sadness, and happiness will serve you well on your healing journey. There will be some feelings you are not comfortable with because they will question your sense of identity.

What does this mean?

If you don't think you're allowed to be scared, you might not even be able to identify some emotions related to being frightened and instead just feel confused. Fear doesn't fit with what you expect of yourself or what you **want** to think of yourself, so you find it hard to know how to describe how you feel.

Naming your emotions is important though because helps you get your needs met. For example:

I feel a bit worried about this, can you talk me through it?

Or I feel lonely, which friend can I call to give me a lift?

Practice makes perfect here. You can find a feelings inventory in the accompanying workbook here

http://jaydiamond.net/abundanceworkbook/

Abandoned by God

For many abuse survivors, in order to get fully on track with your life and create the abundance you truly deserve, a deep core healing needs to take place. But it is a healing you wouldn't think of.

Feeling abandoned by God.

When you have endured horrible circumstances, you rightly wonder how the hell any God could allow such evil in the world. It seems to serve no purpose. Maybe you start to question life itself.

In essence, this thought process is another spiritual gateway, for it is through this quest for understanding that you are led to spiritual teachings on the nature of human suffering and life itself.

This understanding happens only if you come to a point where you stop rejecting life because of the pain and instead become curious about it. So, can you get curious about life?

As you try to make sense of your experiences, you will learn that this life is one of duality. Both the light and the dark exist.

And they ultimately both serve us.

I fought this notion for a very long time; it is often the most difficult of circumstances that shapes the most compassionate of hearts.

The strongest are forged in the fire.

So, let the fire purify you. Use the F word freely – Forgiveness.

Your soul is on a journey that has an agenda separate from the mind, a journey to experience life in its totality, so you can encounter virtues such as strength, compassion, self-direction, spiritual evolvement, forgiveness, and true self-love.

Your soul's journey is different to anyone else's journey, so don't compare your life's journey to anyone else's. It will only cause you pain. Additionally, just because someone looks great on the outside, it doesn't mean they are happy the inside. Hollywood is full of detox centres.

The only way to find out how hard times have served you is to be intentional about it, and ask yourself, "What gifts have come out of this situation; what greatness has evolved in me through this?"

It's not easy, I know, but it's worth it.

When I didn't know how to forgive God for what happened to me, I prayed for life to show me how to heal, instead of asking the usual question, "Why did this happen to me?" I was desperate for peace in my heart, so my ego had to get quiet while I asked to be shown the way to freedom. Then, step by step, I was transformed into a whole new person.

A happier, healthier version of myself.

Many of us are born into this life with beliefs that we are supposed to learn through suffering, and this belief often began lifetimes ago.

But what if you decided right now, that you no longer need to learn about life through suffering?

Decide to choose peace instead.

Decide that you will focus on love, and let love be your guide; even if you don't know how, you will learn.

If you do not feel safe on the earth because of your past, or you resent how life is and resent God - even if it's deep down and you're not fully aware of it - can you see how this would interfere with your ability to create an abundant life? Relationships won't feel safe, feeling sexy won't feel safe, having money won't feel safe, leaving that boring job won't feel safe until you heal this core safety belief.

Our beliefs dictate our behaviour and the circumstances we attract in our life.

What would happen if you decided that instead of ruining your life, your pain is actually your gateway into greater peace, greater truth, and greater version of you - one that gets to choose how you live your life, rather than how others think you should live?

Rather than rejecting your experiences or rejecting yourself, could your pain become a gateway to build a new life for yourself?

Pass through the gateway and don't go back.

Exercise:

Put your hand on your heart, close your eyes breathe five long, slow breaths. Ask to be witnessed by all of life, light a small tealight candle, and declare that from here on out, you will learn about life through love. Hereby release any need to learn about life through conflict, pain, or suffering.

State: "I hereby release any vows of suffering throughout all lifetimes, experiences, planes, and dimensions. I open my heart to the path of love, I breathe love in, and I breathe love out. All is well."

Send your intention into the candle and flame, and let the candle burn all the way out, taking your intention with it.

Summary:

- Pain is your gateway to growth. Use it to build your life now on how you want it to move forward, rather than the past. Then, decide that you will use love to grow from now on.

- Forgive life/ God for your past. Embrace your life and seek the good in life so you can increase your abundance.

- Learn to name your emotions so you can get your needs met.

Go to your workbook for deeper steps into this concept.

SEX

Sex is the holy power of the Divine running through your body.

How does that statement make you feel? Pleased, recognized, and freaked out?

Sex has the ability to heal, empower, and strengthen.

But we don't usually think of it that way. It's more of a need, a fun scratch to itch. Or maybe just overrated.

I feel that we live in a society that is confused and misguided about sex. We generally miss out on its deep healing potency; it is too often used in a way that harms rather than heals.

Sexual energy is the most powerful personal energy we have, but usually we are not taught how to manage this great power. It can feel overwhelming if not channelled appropriately. We teach our young people about the dangers of STI's or pregnancy, but we don't teach them how to say no to sex when they are not ready, or what ready really feels like, especially for a woman who is often more sensitive in nature when it comes to sex.

We don't teach them how to communicate their wants, needs, or fears in a healthy way. We don't teach them about consent and boundaries and how to handle their fluctuating emotions.

That's because most of us as adults don't know how! We just muddled through as a teenager into our adult life, learning as we went along. If we want to see change in the world, we have to start with ourselves.

Many spiritual or manifestation teachers, such as Napoleon Hill in his book, *Think and Grow Rich* (1937), taught that we can use sexual energy to power our creative endeavours and spiritual practices by letting this energy inspire us into movement and motivation. This life force seeks to expand all of life. We can use desire and passion to ignite our business and creative projects!

Because of the strength of sexual energy, many religions over the millennia have taught renunciation.

Renunciation can be defined as being free of lust, craving, and desire, or giving up the 'things' of the world in order to live a holy life. The idea behind renunciation is to make our relationship with the Divine our primary focus and not get distracted by money, sex, and power.

In essence, there is good reason for this teaching; you don't want to get trapped in or obsessed with the material world and miss your spiritual evolution!

However, the way this teaching evolved, and the punishment for not 'following the rules' has led to judgement, repression, and shaming in the area of sex, making sex somewhat taboo. This attitude has relaxed over the last 100 years since the church has less influence over government, and sex is used to sell almost anything these days. Yet, it's still hard to have mature, open, loving conversations about sex and sexuality.

After all, there are hundreds of years of conditioning to overcome.

Many people are comfortable with talking 'dirty,' focusing on the physical aspects of sex, or making a joke of sex in a 'nudge, nudge, wink, wink,' kind of way. But trying to have open, mature conversations that connect both the heart and the body, and regard sex in a loving and sexual way makes people clam up!

They don't know how to do it!

We live in a world that simultaneously objectifies women, and yet somehow expects them to be 'pure' and sexually inexperienced in order to be worthy of love or marriage. Men are conditioned to be proud of their sexual 'conquests,' to not reveal any insecurity about sex, and are expected to *just know* exactly what to do to be a great lover, as if by magic.

This gender conditioning can lead to a pleasurable banging of bodies, if you're lucky, but rarely reveals the deeply connected, ecstatic experiences available to use through sexual union.

The reality is, most of us are not taught how to excel in relationships or sex. We don't recognize the communication that is needed to do this unless we decide as an adult to learn about it. We don't even know that there is much more available to us in our sex lives until we set our egos aside and become willing to learn.

Because we don't know how to ask for what we want or how to have clear boundaries, we may hurt others or be hurt along the way as we explore our sexuality. As a result, we start to close our heart, little by little, especially after a bad break-up. Sex becomes separated from the heart, and eventually it feels as though something is missing.

A series of unconscious and unloving sexual encounters can make us feel confused, lacking confidence, or deeply pained.

In addition, on top of this regular modern-day scenario, many men and women have experienced sexual trauma. When you are sexually abused, groomed, or bullied as a child, teenager, or adult, this trauma can have a far-reaching effect on how you experience sex, relationships, and your own self-worth. These sexual wounds run deep, and I believe they have fractured our society immeasurably, causing us to act out against ourselves or others through uncontrollable anger, self-harming, or addictions.

The experience of sexual trauma can even have a ripple effect, and may affect how well you bond with your children, as well as the fears you pass on to your children; for example, being over-protective, or teaching distorted beliefs to them about how sex, men, and women should be treated. Your pain affects others, not just you.

I believe healing our sexuality is the next frontier in our evolution. This aspect of our lives has been repressed for too long, we need to shed love and light onto it.

We cannot afford to ignore this issue of sex any longer, hoping that it will deal with itself. There is a huge shadow in our collective consciousness related to sex and the sexual trauma many have encountered either directly or indirectly.

Because so many of us carry sexual shame, fear, and disconnection when it comes to our feelings about sex and how we relate sexually to each other, a lack of deep love and satisfaction in regards to sex has become normalized for many.

No. I believe we deserve more. I believe we can have more.

When I discovered Tantra, specifically the left path of Tantra, I found a philosophy that embraces human life and uses that for spiritual evolution and healing, rather than running away from it.

It is easier to go and meditate in the mountains alone to find inner peace than to be slap-bang in the middle of everyday life and know that you are one with God. Go and spend a week with your family and see if you can keep the same equilibrium as a monk in the mountains!

In essence, this is the tantric path; using life itself as a path for spiritual growth, not running away from it, but embracing it to go deeper into healing, acceptance, and love.

It's saying a hearty, "Yes!" to life, and keeping your heart open with all of its experiences.

Although Tantra in the West has become synonymous with sex, it is actually a huge body of teachings. It uses sounds, symbols, movement, purification, breathing practices, and energy to expand the consciousness and connect with the Divine.

A small part of these teachings relate to sexual energy, and they were kept secret for a long time to avoid misuse, because many people misunderstood them.

'White Tantra' is orientated towards spiritual growth and transcending the ego. 'Red Tantra' focuses on the union of the masculine and feminine energies inside and outside the body via an experience of sexual union. 'Pink Tantra' is the middle path of both of these things using sexual energy to open the heart and grow in love and consciousness.

Tantra can be a path that helps us to move through our fears, inhibitions, and insecurities to connect with the Divine/ Higher Self through all of our earthly experiences, by knowing that we are a reflection and creation of divinity.

And our divinity includes our sex.

As we heal our hearts and minds around sex, our interactions with others become sacred, healing, and deeply life-affirming. It is possible to come back to a state of innocence, love, and awe in relation to our sexual selves.

As we embrace the divinity of our bodies, our feelings and our longing for love and the choices we make about sex improve, alongside our self-love, self-acceptance, and self-confidence.

Can you imagine how this world would look if we were all sexually empowered and loving, seeing our bodies as sacred? How would you honour yourself? How would you honour other people?

The world would be transformed!

Although we can't control other people, we do have ownership and responsibility over our own internal world. I believe we are all connected; so as we heal, we give permission and inspiration for others to do the same. As you stand in your power, others will see you and want to know what has changed.

Healing your relationship with sex will create a joyful abundance in your relationships, heighten your ability to receive pleasure, and increase your personal confidence. We are created not just as intellectual or emotional beings, but tactile, sensual beings also. And this is nothing to be ashamed of. We were made for love and sex and joy.

When you have been sexually, physically, or emotionally abused it can cause a huge disruption in your sexual relationships.

A touch that is too gentle or too hard may trigger you to feel sadness or anger, but you don't really understand why. You may find having boundaries difficult and end up in some scary situations that make you feel ashamed or rejected afterwards. You may need sex to build your self-esteem, trying to prove to yourself, over and over, that you are attractive and worthy, and so you constantly seek sex. Conversely, you may find it very hard to trust people at all and so avoid relationships or only bring emotionally unavailable people into your life.

That is how I acted for a long time.

Most of this undercurrent is done subconsciously, and you wonder why you keep ending up in the same kind of situation, even though you thought you were trying to change.

If there is shame related to sex, you very likely have shame about your body. This shame makes you reject your own body which can create numbness in your body and your emotions. Numbness can also appear because you don't feel completely safe in your body - so when feelings of sexual desire arise, other uncomfortable feelings and memories come to the surface at the same time.

This shame can cause you to avoid sex all together.

It's important to realise that when you have been assaulted sexually, especially as a child, your whole perception of and reaction to sex can be distorted. You may have disturbing thoughts, feelings, and memories.

Please know this is a normal reaction to the abnormal circumstances you went through. The mind can create all kinds of thoughts and feelings; not all of them feel good or make sense.

Uncomfortable, odd, or scary thoughts and feelings are not *who you are*, but a *result* of what you have *experienced*. With time and dedication you can heal your mind and heart.

The thing is, when you still have a feeling of shame about past sexual experiences, abuses, or your body, it can cause you to attract partners and experiences that reflect back to you the shame you are hiding inside. This reflection can look like people who treat you badly, dismiss you, give you STI's, shame you for being sexual, or just can't connect with you sexually.

Because we are vibrational beings, what we feel deep down inside sends a message out to life. Other people pick up on it without even knowing it. Therefore a person who feels inadequate inside seems to keep meeting people who treat them badly. This is a universal law: we attract more of how we feel.

When you change the feelings within you, you will instead meet people who are kind and loving towards you, because you have become kind and loving to yourself.

This is why you must love yourself first.

The havoc of unknown shame

Many people see me now as a sexually-empowered and confident woman, but for a long time my sexual relationships were haphazard and disconnected. It was hard for me to really let go during sex, and I didn't often pick men that allowed me to be in my heart or feel safe enough to trust. I was still carrying the pain of the past. I want to share something very personal to me in the hopes that you will understand better how important it is to let go of our shame.

Shame is one of the most damaging emotions we can carry, it creates a heaviness in a person's heart that puts up a barrier to love and draws in more things to be ashamed of. It's a vicious cycle.

Remember, what we believe deep down will keep showing up in our life as a reflection of our internal feelings and thoughts -- whether consciously or below the surface in the unconscious mind.

I sat nervously on the toilet as I craned my deck down to try and see between my legs, but it was too hard to see. I stowed away to my bedroom and got a mirror to work out what the hell it was.

A small fleshy bump, and another and another and another. I felt the first one a few weeks previously but didn't think anything of it, as I didn't look much at 'down there.' An ice-white terror flooded my body like a wave.

Something was wrong with 'it.'

I had seen the slides at school of the penises erupted with lesions and the messiest vaginas I'd ever seen. The message we were given: "some STI's will kill you," rang around my head. I never thought this could happen to me. Like a noose tightening around my neck, I couldn't breathe.

I was usually a boisterous, fun-loving, 13-year old with a smart answer for everything. But now I was silent. I had been so, so careful. How could this happen? It was my second sexual experience; with a guy I was really into but much older than me.

Desperately seeking advice from a friend, I secretly located the clinic and told my mum I was rehearsing after school for the school play. This was an easy lie to believe because I loved dancing and singing so much.

"How many sexual partners have you had? Do you inject drugs?" the nurse asked. "Did you use a condom?"

"Yes," I stuttered through wet eyes. "I did." I was mortified and completely humiliated.

As I undressed quietly, placing one foot and then the other on the cold floor, I pinched myself hard to hold back violent sobs. Panicky and numb, I studied the cracks as I stared at the old ceiling with my legs wide open, jaw tight as the nurse called in the doctor.

I wanted to die.

The nurse was kind, compassionate, and warm. She was so nice to me and I desperately needed that. Then the doctor walked in like a rush of cold air.

"Let's have a look then," he cheerily remarked.

The small bumps were genital warts.

I needed to go back every week to have them treated.

I could make my appointments with the nurse.

Fat tears rolled down my cheeks, as the familiar white fear ripped through my body again. Why was this happening to me? I saw their mouths moving, but I couldn't hear a word. The doctor joked about something or other as I lay helplessly on the bed, with a bright medical light shining directly on my vagina. "Cheer up!" he said as he heartily squeezed my bottom twice and left me with the nurse.

I felt violated and trapped. I didn't need or want my arse happily squeezed while I was stranded on a clinical bed with my legs wide open.

I completely froze in shock. I was ragefully tired of men touching and taking from my body as they saw fit. I wanted to protest, tell him, "Don't you squeeze my arse, you creep. I can't defend myself now!" I felt sick. Why the hell did he do that?! Did the nurse not see?

But I couldn't get a sound out of my mouth as the humiliation of feeling insignificant sank deeper into my body. More helplessness.

More rage to stuff down.

When the nurse told me, the warts came from a virus that might take years to leave my system, the dam broke and so did I. "I'm disgusting, and I'll never get over this," was all I could think. I walked the streets until I could get myself together before going home to talk about the great school theatre show I was rehearsing for.

I only ever told my best friend what was going on.

Before the diagnosis I was always militant about safe sex, which is no bad thing, but as you can imagine, an underlying fear took root about sex and safety.

I believe our physical ailments begin in our emotional body, and warts, metaphysically or spiritually speaking, relate to a belief in ugliness, hate, and lack of self-worth. The truth is, deep in my heart I already felt worthless about myself, and this experience impacted that feeling further.

Confiding this experience to you isn't about blame, or to say that I somehow wanted the experience, or that I deserved it. It's about understanding that our deepest hidden beliefs will show up in our life, one way or another.

Have you ever been at the end of your rope wondering why life just won't let up on you? Or why bad things happen one after another to good people? It seems so unfair.

The problem is, universal law is impartial. It doesn't matter whether you are a selfless volunteer worker, or a greedy tycoon; the universe responds to your core beliefs about yourself and the world, whether you know what these beliefs are or not.

Life showed me how I truly felt inside about myself, and it wasn't sweet.

Before this incident, I desperately wanted to be loved and respected by boys, but deep down thought they were out to get me and weren't to be trusted. My abuse was way in the past, and I didn't think it affected me anymore, as I didn't really reflect on it.

Occasionally, however, I just felt 'dirty,' and remembering the abuse would make me cry with confusion and revulsion. The strange thing was, it would always happen when I felt happy and attractive. My mind linked this feeling with abuse and danger. Happy and attractive and carefree equalled danger to my subconscious mind.

Of course, not everyone ends up with an STI because of past abuse, but I have found with my clients that there is often a lack of self-worth or repressed anger somewhere in the person if they have had this experience.

I want to make this clear once again; this has nothing to do with 'blaming' myself. But I now realise that our minds and bodies are connected, and this knowledge has helped me to understand and heal from my experience.

Life was not trying to punish me; life was merely showing me my hidden pain.

Shame will stop you in your tracks from claiming an abundant life, because deep down you don't think you actually deserve it.

I carried deep shame about those awful months from my teenage years well into my adult life, and I felt a man would never love me if he knew what had happened. Little did I know then, what I know now, how common these experiences are. But because we carry so much shame about them, most people won't ever discuss it. When I eventually did tell someone as an adult, I could hardly speak for crying.

The shame of the past and intimate was tightly locked in my body. I had been stuck in the way my 13-year old self viewed the situation for most of my life -- utter humiliation. But when I finally confessed my past, the world didn't stop. And because I was in good company, I wasn't judged as vile as my trapped 13-year old self viewed me.

Instead, I was just a girl who didn't know what to do, where to go, or how to love herself. I was just a girl who had experienced a bad time; just like many others.

Are there things in your past that have happened, things that you've done, or experiences you've had that you are ashamed of?

If you want to leave Abuse behind and claim your birth right of Abundance, you must decide to let the shame of the past go, once and for all, or it will wreak havoc on your life.

Shame is a silent saboteur.

If you can accept that you did the best you could with what you knew, you will begin to heal. If you understand that holding shame will never change your past, you will be set free. If you can know in your belly that sometimes life feels like it doesn't make sense, but we're all in it together, you will find relief. If you accept that you are born to thrive, not just survive, and that abundance is your birth right, your life will be transformed.

Deciding to love yourself anyway is how you will heal.

Getting a better relationship with sex

So how do you open up to pleasure and reprogram your body and mind?

It's important to know this is a journey, and there is no quick fix. Essentially, you get out what you put in.

Heart

Reconnecting the heart to your sexuality is necessary in order for you to reach the depths of sexual ecstasy, and to feel a sense of deep safety and acceptance. The heights of sexual ecstasy can be reached through focusing on the physical bodies, which is wonderful, but when we dare to connect to the heart, the whole experience is magnified and deepened!

It's very daring to connect your heart to your sexuality.

There are many ordinary people who can't even maintain eye contact during sex because it just feels too intimate, yet they are exchanging bodily fluids with other people!

Having strong discernment about who you share your body with goes a long way to healing your heart. If you sometimes get triggered because of past experiences during sex or sexual acts, you want to be with someone you feel safe to communicate this with, and who is able to be understanding at these times. Whether you are with this person for one night, one month, or an entire lifetime, it is important that you honour yourself by choosing to connect sexually only with people who are respectful, kind, and loving so that your self-esteem builds, not diminishes.

Every choice you make either builds you up or brings you down.

Sex can bring up your insecurities very quickly, so it's important to ask yourself a few questions before engaging with a new sexual partner.

Do I feel safe with this person?

Do I trust this person?

Are they generally a good person?

Is there any kind of crazy that could unfold with this person!?

We forget sometimes to check in with our heart. After early sexual abuse your sex energy may be on autopilot, giving you the green light even though your heart is not sure and not ready. Asking these questions to yourself will improve your boundaries.

A client of mine found she would just automatically take her clothes off and try to wow a new partner sexually very early on, even though her new beau was happy to hang out, talk, and get to know her better. Although she wanted to be loved and valued, she was giving out the message that she didn't want a connection, but that she only wanted sex. This idea was far from the truth, but her body went into autopilot before she knew consciously knew what she was doing.

If this sounds familiar, I urge you to plan ahead of time how you would like your romantic and sexual interactions to play out. Write out scenarios as you would like them to be; write out how you would like to show up, and practice ahead of time. This exercise isn't silly; this is you teaching years of automatic reaction to do something different so you get a different result.

How do you achieve this?

Put your hand on your heart and simply ask:

What would I do if I really loved myself?

When you are still in the process of healing, you can draw partners that reflect back to you the unhealed parts of yourself that feel abandoned, rejected, or like you deserve to be punished.

By asking these questions and deciding on the kind of person you would like to share your sexual self with, plus deciding to act from a place of loving yourself, you will reduce the likelihood of drawing inappropriate partners.

To deepen intimacy with your current partner and to help you stay in your body during sex, eye gazing is a fantastic practice. Sit opposite your partner and hold hands. Maintain eye contact with your partner, looking mainly at one eye for a while (you can't look in both at once) and then the other eye when you need to refocus. Don't let yourself check out or zone out; keep staying present, keep staying focused. Then synchronize your breathing, taking long slow breaths all the way down your body.

Feelings may come up! This is good; this moves you through the layers of fear, taking you closer to your heart. You may want to laugh, but this is a sneaky trick from the mind to distract you. Don't let it.

On the out breath you can think, "I love you," and on the in breath, "I love myself." You want to relax in to this whole process for a good five to 15 minutes. Build up the time, and your heart will blast open.

Having sex after this practice feels deeply connected, safe, and exquisitely sensual. From this place the body can surrender into an abundance of strong orgasms. Hurrah!

Mind

Our mind holds the subconscious beliefs about sex that we don't even know we have. Deep down, we may believe we have to give up our power or manipulate others to have sex. We may not trust the opposite sex, or even like them very much. Or we might believe that sex is the only way to get love.

Conversely, your mind also holds the key to your healing.

The following exercise will help you tune in to the parts of you that are stuck and uncover what you need to do to move forward as it relates to a healthy sex life.

This process involves meeting your inner child. The inner child is the place we all have inside of us that feels like a child or may behave in a child-like way. It's the part of us that feels and reacts.

If, as a child, our needs for love, protection, safety, respect, and guidance were not met, a part of us gets stuck in the past. Then our behaviour comes, not from our adult logical mind, but from the child part of us that never got to process the pain, make sense of it, or move on.

Acknowledging and communicating with your inner child can change your life for the better, for you learn to meet your own needs and love all of the parts that make up 'you,' including the vulnerable, angry, silly, clever, and fun parts.

Your inner child could be happy to connect with you, or angry that you ignored them for so long. Whatever happens, persevere; it will pay off. Because you are connecting with your inner child, do remember that he or she has a **child's perspective** or viewpoint.

You will talk to your inner child about how to heal your sexuality as the adult you are now. Yet, your inner child will have important information for you about how to take care of yourself and what you need in order to move forward in life. Many therapists agree that your inner child needs to get its basic needs of love, appreciation, and attention met before you can become a truly happy, healthy adult, so be open to what unfolds.

In addition, the inner child may talk in a very basic way, so do be open to deciphering its messages if they aren't as clear as you would like.

You will need paper and pen, and you will write down all of your answers with your non-dominant hand. Doing this activates the part of your brain related to feelings, emotional expression, and intuition -- bypassing the analytical mind.

Close your eyes and take a few long, deep breaths.

Relax your muscles and drop your shoulders. Release any tension you feel in your body by breathing into it and softening the muscles.

Imagine you are in a sunny, green field, just breathing in the green and the sunlight. You relax and ask your inner child to come forward. From around the side of a big beautiful tree your inner child appears. Notice how old it is.

Introduce yourself and first ask if there is anything it would like to share with you. Write this down with your **non-dominant hand.** So, if you are right-handed, write the messages down with your left hand, because doing so taps into your feelings.

Explain to your inner child that you are on a healing journey related to sex. Ask your inner child what your biggest blocks are to a happy, healthy sex life.

Then ask, "What do I need to do to I fix this?"

"What support do I need?"

"What support do *you* need?"

Say, "Thank you," to your inner child, and gently open your eyes. If you like, draw a picture of them to help solidify your connection. You can go back to your inner child at any time.

Doing this exercise helps you to tap in to your own inner knowing and points the way to the answers you need to move from Abuse to Abundance in your sex life.

Developing a connection with your inner child will help you to understand what your true needs are and how to look after the part of you that felt abandoned, unloved, or unworthy.

It will help you tune in to the real feelings and fears you have that lie beneath the surface -- the ones that hold you back, but you didn't know were there. Knowledge is power; when you see the truth, you can start to heal. Your inner child will guide you back to love.

Body

For many sexual abuse survivors the feeling of arousal, pleasure, or orgasm has become linked to a feeling of guilt, disgust, or shame. Because there may have been some pleasure felt while the abuse took place, this can set up a lot of confusion in the mind about whether pleasure is good or bad and about whether you are a good or bad person. This confusion can lead to erectile or orgasm problems, or just feeling awful about yourself.

Getting out of your head, out of the self-judgement, and back in to your body is important to allow the body to learn how to be aroused without all of the judgement. We also need to move out of the left brain that likes to control.

You can start to retrain your brain by using gentle touch on your body, clothed or unclothed, and saying positive verbal or non-verbal affirmations to yourself. You can affirm to yourself your name and age and share with your body that you are an adult now. Those hurtful experiences are no longer happening to you.

You might affirm, "It is safe to be sexual now. I am allowed to feel good. My body is my own. I can learn how to enjoy pleasure. I am safe in my body. My body belongs to me, nobody else. I am taking ownership of my pleasure now."

Recognize any emotions that come up and allow them to be released and washed away. If tears come, let them come and let them go. Don't attach to your feelings and don't suppress them either. Let your body let it all go.

Conversely, you may have an abundance of sexual energy and a want to constantly seek sexual experiences. This may be a way to numb other kinds of pain, to seek approval and personal power, or to allow your body to function on autopilot whenever it feels strong sensations. Sometimes masturbation is used as a way to deal with overwhelming emotions.

The high of orgasm can become addictive, and a person may lack discernment in seeking the next high. This may lead to negative relationship patterns that leave you depleted rather than empowered. In this case, asking the questions in the 'Heart' section will help to improve your boundaries. You can use this energy in a healthier way by directing it towards your creativity and motivation for your personal success.

If you have a lot of sexual energy, take responsibility for it. Find healthy outlets that lift you up rather than create drama in your life.

Triggers

If unwanted thoughts, memories, or feelings arise whilst you are having sex or masturbating, there are some things you can do to help shift this uncomfortable experience. However, be aware, this will likely need a deeper therapeutic process if your experiences are very difficult.

Breath, sound, and movement are your best course of action here.

When we are triggered we usually want to push the feeling away rather than deal with it, yet if we can acknowledge the feelings and move through them, their power tends to lessen over time.

If your body becomes tense, or you become numb, breathing deeply and consciously in to your body will help to calm the fight or flight or freeze reaction in the body. Relax your jaw, relax your legs, relax your body.

If you start to float out of your body, or go blank during sex, you can move your body -- your legs, your arms, your head. Open and close your fist to bring feeling and attention to your body. Notice your surroundings, and perhaps add words such as, "I feel like I want to move my legs," or "I need to move," to help you feel present and in your body.

You may want to say, "I need to get up." Then go and change the lighting or go for a walk. You could physically shake your body to shake off the feelings, or say "I want to come back into my body" and have your partner squeeze your arms or kiss you to help you land in your body -- discover what works for you.

It's ok to say: "I need to stop," at any time, to anyone.

You are allowed to ask yourself: what do I need right now? And act on that.

If you feel strong enough, you may wish to gently go into the trigger after you have stopped, paused, and assessed how you feel. Instead of pushing it away, allow yourself to sit and breathe deeply through it. Notice how you feel, and then let it pass.

You may want to scream or punch into a pillow, cry, or even wretch. Keep breathing deeply, keep sending love to yourself, because it's love your body is seeking.

Keep loving yourself through it. Love and acceptance is what will see you through. Making yourself feel bad or blaming yourself will leave you stuck.

It's good to let your partner know what is happening. And you can choose to stay with them or be on your own. Do what is best for you and your partner. It can be hard to explain in the moment, so it's ok to say, "I need some time. I'll tell you later," "I just need a hug," or "I don't feel well right now."

If a trigger comes up that feels very childlike, you can engage in the inner child exercise above at any time. Ask your inner child what they need to heal these triggering experiences.

You can do the same exercise with the trigger itself, as if it were a person trying to get your attention. Go back into the inner child process, and instead, ask the trigger to come forward and tell you what it needs to feel better, and how it is feeling.

Remember to write with your non-dominant hand.

Also, a very powerful process is to plan ahead of time how you would like to handle any triggers that come up for you, and how you would like to let your partner know what is happening. What are your triggers and how do they usually play out? How would you like to show up when this happens? Although this kind of healing may not happen overnight, stating what you prefer to happen does give your mind something to work towards.

It takes practice, and that's okay. Keep on loving yourself through it all.

If it's hard to speak out loud to your partner, you might agree to pinch them, or give a sign if you need to stop. It's good to share all of this with your partner beforehand so they understand that your withdrawal is not about them, but rather about processing your own emotions.

Knowing this, they will most likely to want to support you in your healing journey as best as they can.

Taking care of yourself helps you to claim back your body, mind, and heart as they relate to sex. When you build trust in yourself and open up this deep enquiry into yourself, your nervous system relaxes and anxiety is reduced.

When you have a plan to take care of yourself, there will be more peace within you.

Soul

What has helped me deeply in my recovery is to understand that my soul is on a journey to reveal and experience all aspects of life, both the light and the dark. We live on a planet of duality -- up and down, light and dark, left and right, good and bad. The range of human emotion is vast, and the soul wants to understand all of this human experience.

I decided that I would use my experiences to move to higher ground and be the fuel that drives me towards being my best possible self, rather than staying stuck in my past and wishing it was different. Abuse happened. I survived. I am here. I still deserve the best, and so do you.

Although there is suffering in this life, what I know is that we are not supposed to stay in it, but *evolve through it*. One of the ways I have learned to grow and change is to focus on the journey of my soul.

I believe in reincarnation, that when we die we dissolve back in to the unseen realms, and then re-emerge into a new lifetime, ready for new experiences. The soul seeks to experience virtues as it travels from lifetime to lifetime.

We are here to understand, experience, and express human emotion.

As such, I decided to look for the gifts and lessons on a *soul level* from my sexual abuse. The soul is impartial; it embraces all of life and does not separate things into good and bad in the same way as we do. I asked myself; "What qualities did I develop from this experience; and what positive things did I become? What virtues have I learned?

What good was sparked in me because of this abuse -- not despite it?"

I know this practice sounds counter-intuitive, and most of my clients are very reluctant to do this when I suggest it. It can feel impossible to find anything good from abuse, but I urge you to dig deep, for it will cure some of the desperate need to make sense of such an awful thing.

How?

Because the stories we tell ourselves are incredibly powerful. If you make a decision to **be the hero of your journey and not the victim, it will alter your whole life.**

What if you were someone who was victorious rather than a victim?

What if you learned how to love yourself despite anyone else's actions?

What if you became a more loving, attentive father or mother, not less?

Being sexually abused created an anger in my body to fight for women's rights. Even as a young girl I was sickened by what I saw women go through in our world, and I was perplexed that no one seemed to discuss it at that time; they just accepted it as part of life.

My experiences led me to not simply, 'put up and shut up,' as many girls are taught to do, and this non-compliance contributes to the current paradigm shift on our planet. When I speak up, it gives other girls permission to speak out, to be themselves, to try new things.

In these times, this is an acceptable and occasionally welcome conversation, but just 20 years ago -- before the explosion of social media -- I can assure you it was not.

Later, as I healed at deeper levels through energy healing, plant medicines, and shamanism, I discovered I have been a healer, a witch, a priestess, and a sexual healer for many, many lifetimes. My purpose in this life is to help bring light to the dysfunction around sex on this planet.

Sexual abuse actually catapulted me on a journey of healing that I may not have bothered to take otherwise. I discovered my own healing abilities, and then I started to heal many others. But I could only step into my power on to this path when I had the courage to face my own pain and fear.

This is the story I choose to tell myself, because my story is powerful to me. It doesn't matter if I have proof of all these lifetimes; what matters is how I think and feel about myself, as this story impacts who I am and how I show up in the world.

What is the story you are telling yourself about your soul's journey through this life?

My soul has learned self-sufficiency. I have learned that I am who I choose to be, not what was done to me. My soul learned how to forgive the unforgivable. I have been sparked with deep compassion for others. I really care about people, and they feel safe with me because they trust me. I learned that I am stronger than I thought I was.

I have taken a journey of rediscovering sacred sexuality, and I believe it is time for all of us to really claim our sex as sacred. As I speak openly about these things, others are curious and gain the confidence to start their own healing journey.

Although a part of me still wishes that no one should ever have to go through abuse and discovery, when I decided to look at my life from this perspective, I know I have evolved because of it.

You can also decide to evolve because of your journey. Your decision to tell your story from a different perspective will empower you. You are the director and the actor in your life story, and what started as a tragedy will end in victory. **So tell that story.**

Tell the story of how you *overcame all the odds and still lived brilliantly*. Your current story will shape your future.

If you are still standing; if you have survived, you deserve to acknowledge yourself as the champion you are.

Exercise:

What is the story you are telling yourself about your sexuality? Are you willing to start again and write a new story?

Use your accompanying workbook to rewrite your sexual story.

Summary:

- Sex is holy and so are you.
- Let go of shame or it will wreak havoc over your life.
- You can have a better relationship with sex if you work on it

HEALING BODY HATE

What do you say to yourself when you look in the mirror in the morning?

"Hey you! You look great! Those chins make you look successful! That bed head is kind of like Charlie's Angels!"

Or is it more like, "Ugh! You look tired. Look at that saggy ass. Your hair's a mess!"

Your body hears everything you say.

Many of us spend most of the day listening to the toxic thoughts in our heads, and we are so used to it, we think it's normal. I'm English, and Northern at that, so it's far more acceptable to be self-deprecating than it is to be self-congratulating.

Most people prefer to talk about the bad news, the gossip about what someone did wrong, and the imperfections of others. It is rarer to find someone who typically compliments people, notices what their co-workers do right, or are grateful for all the wonderful things their body does.

"It is no measure of health to be well-adjusted to a profoundly sick society" - Krishnamurti

We have been taught that being ill, anxious, or mildly depressed is something we should take a tablet for, rather than looking inside ourselves to see where we are out of balance. Most of us would never neglect our personal hygiene. We wouldn't dream of going to work without brushing our teeth, putting on clean underwear, or taking a shower.

Yet we feel quite happy to neglect the main thing, besides our body, that gets us through our day -- our mind. Our body and mind are intimately connected, and we often allow the same rotten thoughts to govern our mind, year after year. Studies have shown that negative thoughts actually weaken the body, weaken the muscles, and even weaken the immune system!

Our unloving thoughts are making us sick!

Here's the thing: you don't have to believe everything you think. Every thought you have isn't the truth. There can be old stories, messages from TV, magazines, movies, family, and even old school teachers that show up in your head as your own thoughts.

How would life be if you decided only to entertain pleasant thoughts, and no longer gave nasty thoughts the time of day?

"Thoughts are things, and powerful things at that." - Napoleon Hill

Your body has its own memory of all your lived experiences in its cellular structures and tissues, both the good and the bad. It also hears what you say about it.

To move from Abuse to an Abundance of love and health in your physical body, you have to continually remind yourself of two things:

1. Your body is home to your soul
2. Your body is the way you experience life.

Because it is the home of your soul, loving and honouring your body is paramount to your healing.

Your body is the vehicle through which you experience the world. It's how you hug, kiss, pick up your kids, dance, sing, and play. It's part of your human experience, and to truly feel like you belong to life, you need to accept the body you have.

Learning to love your body is the process of lovingly accepting yourself exactly as you are, right here, right now. That's why it's so important.

Refuse to speak badly about your body.

Refuse to think badly about your body.

Instead, re-frame your thoughts and compliment your body. However, don't outright lie to yourself and say, "I love my belly!" if you still feel like you hate it, because your mind will really push back.

Instead, use phrases such as:

I'm open to the possibility of loving my belly.

I'm grateful for my arms, as it means I can hug.

I am learning to love my tummy.

I am becoming happier every day.

I am grateful for my thighs, they are strong!

When you focus on the benefits of your body, you build new, positive associations with it. By using words like learning, becoming, and possibility, you teach the mind how to accept positive words, without saying, "Oh no, you're a liar!"

When these affirmations feel comfortable, you might progress to, "I really do love my cute tummy!"

When you change way you think about life, the life you think about will change. Let's make this change for the better.

If you have lived through emotional, physical, or sexual abuse, it's important to show your body more love, not less. It needs your affirmation, your kindness, your acceptance.

Body issues are a big problem for many of the people who come into my group online programs because we can easily blame our bodies unnecessarily. The good news is, we really **want** to feel good in our body and with some effort, we can do just that.

Our bodies are such miracles! We don't have to watch over the lungs, heart, blood, or liver to keep them working; it's all completely automatic. But we don't tend to look at the body as miraculous. Our society is obsessed with portraying 'perfect' (according to this culture) bodies, and this idea really does reflect how, as a society, we value what's on the outside more than the inside.

It's only in recent years that we are starting to see some plus-sized, older, and even Down syndrome models on the catwalks and magazines, but they are still few and far between.

I found that many women will openly talk about what they don't like about their bodies, from cellulite, feeling fat, uneven breasts, or 'bingo wings.'

However, many men have these struggles too, concerning their weight, not feeling masculine enough, or penis size. It's just not as socially acceptable for men to talk about these issues because they are told not to be weak, or that they have no right to say anything because they don't have it as bad as women. This argument is crazy; life's not a 'feel-bad' competition.

When I started holding women's circles, I found that many women really don't like how their vaginas look and would never dream of taking out a mirror to look at themselves. The vagina is referred to as 'down there' or 'my downstairs' and it freaks them out to talk about it.

If I were to propose that you could love your genitals, and make friends with your genitals - would you find this a ridiculous notion? Would you feel anxious, or just turn away from such a silly idea?

Making friends with and learning to accept and love your own sex organs goes a long way to full body self-acceptance. It helps you to honour and recalibrate yourself as a sexual being. It is a strong indication of body love. Your genitals are part of your body and are just as sacred and beautiful as everything else.

It's the 21st century, and most women are still embarrassed to talk about their monthly period or admit when their body needs rest. We still feel we have to keep up the image of perfection.

How can you fully let go in the bedroom when you reject your sexual organs? How can you believe in someone else's adoration of you when you reject yourself? Even if the love is there, you probably won't believe it.

I invite you to start practicing radical acceptance of yourself. We fear we won't drop the weight, or be as attractive if we don't beat ourselves up about what we don't like, but this simply isn't true.

Making the declaration, ***"I've decided to love myself anyway!"*** will lead you to be motivated by love instead of fear.

And love feels a whole lot better.

Weight

We may use excess weight to act as a buffer to the outside world and our own feelings. We may use being underweight as a way to control the feelings too. Weight problems that cause you to feel awkward in your body are rarely just about too much or too little food.

For those with excess weight, as they diet, exercise, and drop a few pounds, they often feel great at first, but at some point, they stop losing weight and the weight goes back on.

Sometimes excess weight is maintained by the beliefs that underpin what you associate with different levels of weight. If you cannot shift the weight, there are usually hidden beliefs that make you feel safer or more accepted at a certain weight. Common misbeliefs relate to not feeling safe if you feel you are attractive, that your family and friends will reject you if you're slim, and the belief that if you're successful, life will change, and you don't like change.

When you criticize and are jealous of others with the kind of great body you want, you expect others to act in a similar way towards you. You want to fit in with friends and family and not be rejected by them because you have grown into a healthier, happier body, so you subconsciously sabotage your own progress.

Conversely, if you believe you are not loveable unless you are very slim and extremely beautiful, you may forever find fault with yourself and never be satisfied with your body, regardless of how pretty and slim others say you are. You still hate your body, and never feel good enough.

Issues can arise if you had life difficulties at a certain weight. If at a particular weight you lost your father, or you were in a difficult relationship; as you shift the weight these feelings can start to rise again.

Your fat cells hold memories and store feelings to protect you. As you release layers of fat, the toxins and the feelings stored at that layer will come up too. This is when we just start to lose the motivation we once had. Knowing all of this can help you to keep moving forward.

Daily affirmations can be helpful here, such as:

It is safe to have a great body,

I am always loved.

I have decided to love myself at every shape and size.

I can process my emotions and still love my body.

I don't have to be perfect to be loved.

I have found EFT (emotional freedom technique) tapping is a great tool to help reprogram negative beliefs, so I teach this in my online program.

A Japanese researcher called Dr Emoto, stunned the world when his experiments on water found positive and negative words had an effect on the molecular structure of the water. Positive words, made symmetrical crystalline structures in the water, and negative words made the structure disorganized and chaotic.

Your body is made up of 70% water! Like I said, your body is listening to your every word.

Bless your body and bless your food. "Thank you," and "I love you," said with true intent are simple and powerful blessings.

Yoni and lingham love

Having a deep and loving relationship with another requires a deep and loving relationship with yourself. Healing means embracing who you are, what you look like, the scars you have, the mistakes you've made, and the past you've lived.

This healing is true acceptance. You don't deny the past, it's just you're no longer controlled by it. Importantly, you stop needing the past to change for you to be happy. True acceptance is deciding to be happy anyway. You can see the gift and the lessons in every experience, even if you'd prefer to have not had that experience.

When there is self-acceptance, you make decisions based on the present, not the past. This means you make far better decisions for yourself each and every day.

Because the body has a memory all of its own, when you've experienced abuse you might need to reset your physical body, as well as the spiritual and emotional body.

A woman holds a lot of emotion in her womb and vagina. A man can hold a lot of tension in his testicles, anus, and penis. We all tend to unconsciously constrict our anus when we're in fight or flight mode, and stressed. It's just the body's physiology at work, but it can mean we hold unknown tension there for a long time that spreads to our back, legs, and genitals.

For a heterosexual woman who *receives* a man physically in to her body, she may take in their stress and tension too, as she is in receiving mode. Some say this energy stays around for a few days or weeks, but in extreme circumstances I believe it can stay for years. I have worked with many women who have energetic ties to past partners or past sexual experiences in their womb. Somehow, the energy of the past partner is still with them and they can't fully move on.

Yoni (vagina) and lingham (penis) massage when done by the right trusted therapist can release years of stored tension, emotional blockages and the memory of past trauma stuck in the body. Yoni and lingham are ancient Indian Sanskrit words.

The first time I had a yoni massage, I cried and cried as years-old panic was released from the internal tissue of my vagina.

The cervix also holds a lot of trapped emotion, and many women are shocked to find that many parts of their vagina are numb inside, they have become shut down internally, not trusting life or partners after being hurt. With time, care, and attention the inside of the vagina can be re-enlivened.

Prostate massage (inside the anus) is often part of the lingham massage, and for men particularly, is incredibly healing. Many men are shocked at the sheer level of rage, emotion, and stress that is relieved from this practice alone. Years' worth of repressed emotion can be released revealing a happier, more relaxed man.

Many heterosexual men or men who have been abused can feel very resistant to this idea; however, I have seen it have deep transformational effects. Of course, always find a practitioner you trust and feel safe with.

Even a masturbation practice where you consciously give yourself lots of love, care, and positive affirmation can have a positive effect on your self-esteem.

In ancient traditions the archetype of the feminine was revered and worshipped. Her womb was revered as the portal that it is between earth and heaven. Woman was respected as the vehicle through which our divine souls enter the planet; and her menstrual blood, with its life-giving stem cells, was truly honoured.

All over the world there were temples, statues, and altars dedicated to the feminine, but as patriarchal structures rose, these temples, along with their priestesses, were systematically obliterated.

It's no wonder many men and women don't see the pussy as something to be revered and honoured as the temple of life that it is.

Woman: the holy grail is your womb, the keeper of life.

Man: you carry the spark of God in your semen.

How would you show up for yourself, in your relationships and in your sex life if you held these beliefs? How would you treat your awesome, miracle of a body?

Ladies, who do you let inside? Any passer-by with a sweet word? Is your body a place for others to dump their stress, leaving you depleted and empty?

Or do you only allow those with devotion and honour to enter your temple?

Guys, are those you connect with people who add something to your life, or do they cause drama and chaos? Do you respect and honour that spark of God that creates life from you?

When we have experienced violation, we can either lock the temple doors for good, or forget to guard the entry, because we forgot the temple is holy. It's time to remember who you are. You have the choice to recreate yourself as you wish to be now. You are a creator of your future, not a prisoner of the past.

For me personally, to be in my full power as a woman it has been imperative that I heal the relationship I have with my vagina and womb, so that I can remember my temple is holy, and treat myself as such.

I created an easy downloadable workshop so anyone can access this kind of healing and self-honouring.

Recalibrating the body as a safe place

In one Ayahuasca journey, the plant spirit helped me to unplug the power that memories of my abuse had over me. I rewired my brain and released trapped energy to reduce the emotional charge associated with these events. When I breathed through the tension and stayed present with the fear instead of pushing it away, eventually the fear subsided.

When the emotional charge of our past is processed and released, there is more energy available to create the life you do want, instead of subconsciously spending mental energy pushing away thoughts and feelings you don't want.

I could see myself as an eight-year old girl lying on that bed. And in my mind's eye, I saw myself as an adult gently lie down behind my childhood self. I guided my inner child to put her hand over her yoni, and I, the grown-up healing woman, rested my hand on top of hers.

In real time, during this ceremony, I lay fully clothed, with my hand over my yoni, connecting with the energy of myself as a child. In my mind and heart, I was connected to that little girl, that eight-year old me, and giving her all the comfort and love she needed. I let her feel loved and cared for.

I changed the feelings that got trapped in the past, by giving myself love in the present, and by sending love back to myself at eight-years old.

I called in love, healing, and white light to reset the energy and cells of my vagina and womb to heal them from abuse, rape, and the many other unloving sexual experiences I have had over the years. As I held this intention, a powerful light coursed through me.

It was time, **"To be in, and love wholeheartedly, your woman's body,"** said the medicine.

I felt different; something had changed. As I looked inside of my body, not with my physical eyes, but with my internal sight, I saw a clear, happy, radiant womb. I reclaimed my vagina.

Reset, reboot, and renew.

Tears rolled as I remembered the times over my life I had betrayed my own heart to seek affirmation or love from men; the times I was preyed on when I was weak.

I grieved for the loss of my innocence, grief I didn't know I had, yet I knew I was ready to let it all go.

Reset, reboot, and renew.

I am proof that it is possible to reverse the pain of the past and restore your heart to love. This restoration was an utterly life-changing gift.

"The womb is a sacred place," said the Ayahuasca spirit. My womb deserves to be free of fear, anxiety, and past conditioning, to grow a new life.

I knew I was creating a better start for my future children.

Exercise:

You can create your own visualization to revisit yourself at a painful point in the past. Was there a time when you didn't feel good about your body, appearance, skin, or weight? Take yourself there in a relaxed meditation, perhaps by listening to some calming meditation music.

As your wise, adult self, go back and give your younger self all the love and reassurance that you needed at that painful point in the past.

What does your younger self need to hear to feel better?

Tell your younger self what they need to hear to feel better. Tell them about all the great things you have now achieved in your life, and share with them all the great qualities that you see in them.

Give yourself comfort and breathe love into your body.

When you have done this, you will find you start to feel more comfortable in your body, though you may need to go back more than once and keep filling up your younger self with love and self-assurance.

Summary:

- Make friends with your body by refusing to criticize it. Use kind words and positive affirmations.

- Bless your body and bless your food.

- Learn to love your genitals. They are part of your body too!

Money

When there has been abuse to children or teenagers, it creates a trauma or disconnect in their primary relationships, sense of security, or sexuality. The first and second chakras get out of balance, and these two chakras also relate to money. The root (first) chakra relates to your childhood and issues of security, and the sacral (second) deals with relationships, puberty, sexuality, and creativity (creativity relates to our ability to manifest things).

The chakras are energy centres in our body that we can't see but are there; this is what the ancient yogis and Chinese medicine taught us. Each energy centre relates to a stage of development, moving from basic security matters to higher spiritual experiences.

The ability to feel secure at the root chakra includes financial security. You may not feel safe, or trust that all will be well if you have too much money. There may be more fear attached to money than desire.

Remember, the mind will always do more to avoid pain than it will to gain pleasure.

If you weren't nourished as a child you might hold the belief that there is 'not enough' in the world, and this becomes reflected in your financial situation.

Even if by other people's standards you have enough, you will always feel like you don't, or that your abundance will run out.

These beliefs often aren't rational, so the conscious, thinking mind doesn't see them.

The 'I'm not enough' belief and money

One of the core issues I find beneath the surface of almost all people I meet is, 'I'm not good enough.' This belief might concern having the relationship of their dreams (It failed before; it will fail again -- it must be me), stepping into their life purpose (Who am I to think I can do amazing things? I don't have the qualifications; I feel like a fraud), or having great wealth (That's for someone else. It can only come through hard work, and I don't want to work so hard. I can't have it all).

When a person has an abusive background this 'I'm not enough,' belief can be strongly hard-wired and cause sabotage in his or her money situation, as well as many other areas.

Working on reversing this belief will serve you well. What happened in your past does not dictate your future. Each and every one of us is worthy and deserving of great abundance as wealth.

The 'I'm not good enough' fear is the voice that tells you that you will never make it. It says you can never be as good as those you are comparing yourself to, so why bother putting in 100%? There are many people who are at the top of their game but still suffer from, 'I'm not good enough,' and it drives them to overwork, never feeling satisfied, and various addictions to deal with the stress of feeling inadequate no matter what they achieve. This results in being stuck in the endless hustle of chasing more, rather being open to receiving the universe's stream of abundance.

We usually try to suppress the 'not good enough' voice but suppressing it won't make it go away. The real trick is to make friends with this voice. It is a fear response that wants to keep you safe. We can be afraid of both failure and success, as with either result, our life may change.

Exercise:

Close your eyes for a few moments and feel that fear, the voice that says you're not good enough to have what you want.

Ask the fear what it is trying to protect you from.

Then ask the fear how you can feel safe and still get what you want.

Write down your findings.

Flowing sexual energy and money

A person with blocked sexual energy tends to have issues with money.

I found during my own healing journey that the more I allowed myself to have pleasure of all sorts, including sexual pleasure, my abundance increased. I could let more of the goodness in life in to my personal world.

It's not that I didn't enjoy sex, but rather there were emotional blockages that limited how much pleasure I could contain and how safe I felt at a deep level in my personal and sexual relationships. These were issues I wasn't even aware of for a long time.

This is why when you commit to your healing process, you see results across your whole life. You may find developing new trust in your friendships opens up more trust in your work life.

Sexual abuse, in particular, has a sneaky way of interfering with many areas of your life, not just sex, because of the beliefs and fears that arise from that experience.

So, I could *make* money, but couldn't *contain* it or keep it for long. A household item would break, an unexpected bill would arrive, or a not-to-be-missed, *yet expensive,* opportunity would come up. I became used to having just enough to get by, and this was a theme that ran across my life. I didn't put my needs first.

A flowing sexual energy is a free-flowing energy of desire. Allowing yourself to feel desire without needing to control the outcome is what magnetises you towards that which you wish to have. Sometimes we are too afraid to want something, in case we get let down.

The second chakra rules pleasure and receptivity of pleasure, so when this chakra is open and balanced, we feel free to receive good in our life. We feel worthy of having more than enough, we feel worthy of being in overflow, creativity, money, and abundance.

As I mention in the chapter about sex, sexual energy is a motivator and a creative force. Allow yourself to feel the desire of the life you would like to create, allow yourself to build pleasure in your body, without having to quickly suppress it or release it with an orgasm.

You can even build sexual desire in your body and meditate on that which you would like to create to manifest it more quickly. Some even say money is orgasmic energy in form, as it is a means to create things. Therefore, money is attracted to flowing sexual energy.

When we feel sexy and abundant, we attract more of it! Yet when we feel down and worried about money, we seem to have more things to worry about!

Allow yourself to have more pleasure in your life. Release your blockages to sex and relationships and watch your abundance increase. Build your own internal sense of self-worth and self-pleasure by making yourself feel good. I worked with coaches and healers to do this and got clear on what my underlying negative beliefs were, so I could change them. I also use music, dance, and self-pleasure to pour love into myself.

Vibration

Money is simply an energy like any other. Everything is essentially made up of energy at its deepest level. We are like radio transmitters giving and receiving energy all the time. So, what you believe about money is what life will transmit back to you. Therefore, it's important to get in a right relationship with money if you want to flow in your life.

If you don't like handling money or are always complaining that you have to chase it, then money will always be hard to keep hold of. Having money in your account is not simply about your qualifications, your work ethic, or good financial guidance. It's more about your beliefs about money, your self-worth, and your mindset.

If your honest belief is, "Well if someone else has done it, so can I!" and your mindset is, "I'll get the help I need to make it possible!" then the world is your oyster.

The truth is, the universe itself is abundant.

Just look at Mother Nature and all of her gifts - the water, the air, the food, the land. We are set up to be abundant. The problem is we are born into a world that tells us there is not enough to go around. That someone must win and someone must lose. Perhaps our family taught us we will never have enough, and we believed it. But it simply isn't true.

The universe itself is abundant.

Get that idea down in your spirit. No matter what happened in the past, decide this belief will be true for you now so you can open up to the goodness that life wants to give you.

The real problem is how much abundance we will allow into our lives due to our beliefs. This is the law of the universe: we have free will. We can believe in abundance or we can believe in lack. It's our choice. When we believe in lack, we are never satisfied no matter how much we get. When we believe in abundance, we are grateful for all the small things as well as the large, and we feel good about life.

Perhaps you've had unpleasant experiences in the past, and you have always felt like you won't have enough. This thought still does not have to dictate your future from here on out. What happened in your past was created from what you knew then, the thoughts you had then, the life you had then.

When you clean up your thinking and feelings about money, what happens in the future can and will change.

There are many, many successful people who had a very hard start in life. They made it, and so can you. Fill yourself up with inspirational videos, stories, books, and memoirs of successful people who overcame adversity. Command your brain to understand that your adversity works to your advantage. Troubles make you savvy, compassionate, and motivated. If you've overcome hard times in the past, you certainly have the wherewithal to learn about and master how to allow money into your life now. Not everyone needs a million dollars, but you do deserve to always have more than enough.

Jim Carey had to drop out of school when he was 15 to support his family. Now, he is a household name, due to his extensive film career.

Oprah Winfrey suffered awful abuse at home and at age 14 got pregnant, then gave birth to a child that passed away. She is now an international media personality with numerous businesses, and she helps millions of people.

Jay Z couldn't get any record labels to sign him. He made his own label, and the rest is history.

Malala Yousafzai is renowned world-wide. She was shot in the head after standing up to the Taliban in Pakistan and demanding that girls be allowed an education. She survived, became a children and women's-rights activist, and won a Nobel Peace prize.

Your past does not define your future. No matter how bad it is now, your future can always change.

With practice, you can gain control over your mind and thoughts, so when you catch them going down the rabbit hole of worry, stop and ask yourself:

So, what if life did turn out all right after all?

Play that new story out in your mind instead. Doing so retrains the way your mind goes on autopilot towards worry. Some argue this tactic is silly and useless.

But, those of us who use it know worry is like riding a rocking horse to nowhere. It doesn't take you where you want to go, it just gives you something to do. So be practical. Make plans, budgets, savings, and debt repayments, then go back to positive thoughts that give you hope. Allow yourself to feel good.

Why? Because how you feel is what you transmit to life. Always choose thoughts that feel better when it comes to money if you want it to flow in your life. This choice takes practice, of course. The secret to all manifestation is making feeling good within your first priority. When you feel off balance, this is the first thing to do because we make the best decisions when we feel good.

Have you ever made a decision in haste or anger and regretted it afterwards? It's because you were focused more on fear than love.

"Let your alignment (with Well-Being) be first and foremost and let everything else be secondary. And not only will you have an eternally joyous journey, but everything you have ever imagined will flow effortlessly into your experience. There is nothing you cannot be or do or have—but your dominant intent is to be joyful. The doing and the having will come into alignment once you get that one down."

- Esther Hicks

Do not underestimate the state of your internal feelings and its relationship to how money shows up in your life. Misery loves company, but money loves happiness. That's why you get more and more when you're 'on a roll!'

If you're serious about changing your views stay away from music, films, tv programs, and people who complain about lack of money, or have negative messages about money; especially while you are retraining your brain to believe in abundance. These things influence your thoughts, and you want to be full of good feelings about money.

Gratitude

Many have taught about the importance of gratitude as a way to magnetise to you more things to be grateful for. This ideology is also true of money. When you send out the vibration of gratitude in regards to money and your material life, you tell the universe you are happy and are open to more. You tell the universe that you believe in abundance rather than lack.

You can tell the universe you are open to more goodness by writing out ten things you are grateful for and why each morning. This sends the transmission of abundance out, so abundance can flow right back to you.

When you receive money of any amount, really feel the gratitude in your heart. When you pay bills, feel that gratitude of having heat, light, clean water, and a roof over your head. Feel gratitude that you have the money to pay that bill, rather than begrudging it. Feel grateful that you have a phone and access to comforts that many others in the world do not. Keep finding new things to say thank you for. Continue expressing gratitude so you can tip the scale from feeling lack to feeling abundance.

It all starts with how you feel; then the manifestations occur.

Money is just paper. What we do with it reflects who we are. If you want to take advantage of people, you will do more of that. If you want to love and assist people, you will do more of that. It is your choice.

We can get caught up in the perils and unfairness of the world, thinking, "How can I dare to be abundant when so many other are going without?" My reply to this question is; can you ever be poor enough to help someone else get out of poverty?

Can you ever be ill enough to cure another's disease?

For you to go without adds no value to someone else's struggle. Overcoming your problems inspires others to know they can do the same for themselves.

I believe when good people prosper, they do more good. Do well, so you can do more good! That's what this world needs right now, people who care and will make a difference. Make your money vision larger than just meeting your own personal needs. How would you be of service if money wasn't an issue?

You can start right now from where you are.

Being of service is one way to move from Abuse to Abundance; you use your plenitude to make a difference in other people's lives. It can be as simple as a regular £2 donation to a children's charity, or fund raising for a women's shelter or an abuse helpline for men. You could do wonderful things with money when you are in abundance and overflow.

You deserve it. We all do.

Money exercises:

Get your notepad out and have a look at your money story. How do you really feel about money in this world? What do you dislike? What do you like? What negative beliefs do you have?

Just start brainstorming. You might see thoughts like: money corrupts, rich people are greedy, people change when they become wealthy, if you earn a lot, it just gets taxed anyway.

Take a good look; because these are the beliefs that keep you apart from the abundance you desire.

Now write your money story as you would like it to be. Write your story with emotion about overcoming adversity and how you show up in your life at 100%. What are your beliefs and actions? What assistance do you get? What great things can you do with lots of money, and what causes would you champion and donate to? What difference will you make in this world?

Read your new money story to yourself each morning and train your brain for success.

Summary:

- The belief, 'I am not enough,' will sabotage you

- Your pleasure and sexual energy are linked to your finances. Increase your capacity for pleasure to increase prosperity.

- Gratitude and vibration are everything. Make it your intention to feel positive as much as possible about money. Watch your thoughts!

THE COURAGE TO BE INTIMATE

When you are really hungry, you will eat junk food that you know makes you feel bad. You will snack on someone else's candy bar and dig out the old bag of nuts you left at the bottom of your rucksack.

When you get used to eating junk food, you get used to the quick fix of an instant hit of the higher levels of sugar and salt. You don't even feel like looking at a healthy plate of protein and vegetables. Even though you are getting fat and feel sluggish, you reach for the junk food because it's what you know and what you like, and you've become addicted to it. Even when your health starts to deteriorate and you have to visit the doctor, you carry on. It's only when things get really, really bad that you finally wake up, and say, "Hey, something needs to change." But by this time, you are so ingrained in your bad habits, you don't know how to make good habits anymore.

What's worse is almost all of the people you know eat various forms of junk food, so their advice on how to get healthy doesn't seem to last long because they don't really know how to get healthy either. Because you are so unfit, the whole process seems too overwhelming, and you resign yourself to believing, 'that's life.'

The same mistakes happen in love.

We are born into a world that largely doesn't know how, and therefore doesn't teach us how to create and maintain healthy intimate relationships. We pick up bad habits from our parents or community, and we just do our best on limited or erroneous information.

If we have been hurt on purpose or by accident by family, friends, and past loves, we gradually build up a hard shell around us to protect ourselves. The shell keeps us a little safer to some extent, but it also limits how much love we can receive through the shell, and how much love can get out. Because everyone else has this shell, it feels quite normal.

But we are not born this way.

Babies and small children are so exquisitely joyful to be around because they haven't formed their shell yet. They just give and receive love freely and with joy, and their simple laughter can light up your whole day. They are carefree and present in experiencing how they feel now. They are not too worried about whether you will reject them if they come and play with you, and they are not dwelling on the kid who wouldn't share their toys with them last week.

The shell is a barrier of fear, and it influences our thoughts and actions. We fear being hurt or judged, so we paint the shell with the image we want to project out into the world, so that people will like us. We can make the shell very handsome, very slim, or very clever, but it is still just the shell, and it's full of the ways we have learned to protect ourselves from being hurt.

Most of the time, when two lovers meet, they encounter the outer shell.

When we relate to another person through our shell, we interpret our partner's actions through the fears of our own outer shell. This may make us act passively, so they don't leave us; controlling, so they don't leave us; or aggressively, so they will just go ahead and leave us because that is what we expect anyway.

We may display a variety of emotions in order to feel safe and respected.

When the two outer shells between partners meet, we may become disappointed when we realise that they are not all they painted themselves out to be. Gradually the mask slips as they can't keep up the perfect picture forever.

The best way to attract the right partner for you, is to work on loving yourself first, by filling up your own heart with love and being and expressing your true self, instead of the painted outer shell.

There is someone in this world who wants someone just like you, but they won't be able to see the real you if you pretend to be the perfect outer shell.

If we have been emotionally, physically, or sexually abused in the past, we learn that it's not safe to trust and that people let you down. This belief vibrates in your outer shell and sends the message out to life, "It's not safe to love!" This image is what life reflects back to you like a mirror in the people you meet, and you again feel that love is not safe

But if you believe in love more than you believe in fear, you can tip the balance. If you learn to fill up your own heart with love, this will overflow, and you will start to attract people who reflect this love back to you. Your own shell will be filled with love, and gradually it will soften and dissolve.

But how?

1. Watch your thoughts, expectations, beliefs, and reactions to love.

Write down your fears about love, so you can see clearly what you are dealing with. What do you secretly expect a partner will do? What do you believe about love and about men, about women? When you are dating or in love, what are the fears that rise up?

Then ask yourself is this fear true? Is it always true? Or is it true for you, but not always true for others?

We can tell ourselves that love doesn't exist, yet others believe it does. Which would we prefer to believe?

Once you tell the truth on the fears that come up, you can start to challenge your usual reactions. You can practice asking questions instead of simply making assumptions that your initial belief about a person or situation is always right. You can practice responding to challenges in a different way so get you a better outcome. This will soften the hard, outer shell and pave the way for true, intimate, lasting connection.

2. Pour love into yourself.

A person that loves themselves draws more love to them. Get out a notepad and list the ways you would love a partner to treat you, speak to you, and feel about you.

Then treat, speak, and feel about yourself the way you desire to be loved.

The funny thing about life is when you go begging with an empty cup no one wants to share; but when your cup is full others will add to it in Likewise, when you believe you are empty, no one wants to pour into you as it never feels like enough, yet when you carry the belief you are full, others are drawn to give to you

Why? Because what you believe is either pushing away or pulling towards you what you want. Once again, I remind you, it all starts inside of you.

Instead of making your partner your primary source of love, make yourself your primary source of love and allow your partner to add to your cup. This means that whatever decisions your partner makes, whatever fears they experience inside their shell, your cup is always full.

To move from Abuse to Abundance in love, you need to detox from your old beliefs and behaviours, and train yourself to have healthier beliefs and habits. It is not enough to just say, "I love myself," you have to act in ways that show this love.

If you really loved yourself, how would you act; who would your friends be; how would you spend or save your money; who would you allow into your life?

This detox from negative beliefs is like a training program that takes practice. You may not be perfect at first, but with time and effort you will attract more and more love in to your life; the love you truly deserved all along.

Not everyone will be happy for you when you start to dismantle the shell.

They may get upset that you are daring to be different. Your bravery reminds them of their own fear, and they don't like it. Even though you are not judging them, they feel judged. This impression is because they secretly judge themselves when they see you trying to make your world a better place. They may even try to sabotage your progress to prove that they are right and you are wrong, insisting that the only safe place is in the shell.

When you allow toxic people in your life, whether a friend or a lover, it changes you for the worst. You become someone you don't want to be because of their influence, and those bad habits and fears you develop can take years to undo. Be aware of the people who help you grow and the people who drag you down; avoid the latter. You are allowed to leave toxic people behind or keep your distance from them, especially when you are practicing a new version of yourself.

Put more energy and attention into people and things that make you feel good. Turn down offers from toxic people and walk away from gossip. You don't have to make any big declarations; just make the changes you need to make.

Our love relationships are challenging because they stir up fear in the outer shell. The shell that you built to protect you feels threatened by a love it fears may be taken away, and you will begin to see all the unhealed fears float to the surface as the shell fights to protect you from love. It sees love as leading to pain. The deeper the love, and the more honest and real you are in your relationship, the more fears that will arise.

If you hide behind the shell, perhaps only one or two fears will arise, but if you peek out from behind it, so that your real self can meet your partner's real self, the shell will guard itself against any possible pain. All of the old fears you thought were put to rest will suddenly reappear for your appraisal. This point is when most of us snap back and retreat into the shell, but it is, in fact, a huge opportunity to heal the wounds of the past by enquiring whether these beliefs are really true now.

It takes enormous courage to brave real intimacy with another human being and allow yourself to be seen for all you are: the tender, the awesome, and the vulnerable. And it also takes courage to allow your partner to be all of they are and just accept them for it.

We know it feels amazing to be emotionally connected to a partner, yet when you've experienced heartbreak, the fear of being hurt again can be torturous. That fear causes you to act in ways that sabotage your relationship by not allowing you to open up, in an effort to avoid emotional pain.

We fear we'll lose our freedom, get stuck with the wrong person, or be abandoned once they get to know the 'real me.'

So, up pop the sabotaging behaviours: overworking, searching for fault in your partner, focusing on the negative, picking someone who isn't emotionally available, withdrawing, lying, keeping secrets, withholding affection, clinging when the partner tries to be independent, drinking, being emotionally aloof, or some other negative reaction.

We may secretly think, "If I don't fully invest, I won't be hurt so much." But real love is the balm that heals all wounds.

When you have been conditioned from an early age that you have to work hard for love when it is offered freely to you, you won't trust it, and so you push it away.

You can be in a relationship or have sex with someone but not necessarily be intimate. Intimacy is an emotional closeness and openness. This emotional closeness increases as the outer shell decreases. Intimacy is feeling seen, heard, loved, and accepted on a deep level. It's is the kind of connection we crave, but rarely find because of the shell.

In my workshops and one-on-one work with couples, I guide them through simple practices to get out of their heads and into their hearts again, to feel real intimacy. The simple practice of gazing into another's eyes can be incredibly difficult for some people, bringing up tears and uncomfortable feelings. We rarely hold another's gaze for more than a few seconds, but when we do, something magic happens.

The shell starts to soften, and we see the person before us from our heart instead of through all the beliefs in our head. We connect on a heart level, and without words, we feel accepted and can just 'be.' No trying to please, no mask, no shell. Someone can feel so much closer to their partner simply by letting go of their shell and allowing their partner to just be.

When we share our deepest feelings with another it creates intimacy, but that closeness requires vulnerability and trust. This intimacy, of course, is built over time, and with a person who proves themselves to be genuine. It is still damn scary though! We are afraid to look weak, insecure, unsure, not perfect somehow.

The mind says no way! They will hurt me! I can't do it!

Of course, intimacy is not telling all your deepest wounds and hurts to every person that comes along in an effort to tell the truth. We must always use discernment. There is a difference between sharing how you feel and dumping all of your emotions on someone.

The path of the heart is to practice being authentic; sharing how you feel, sharing that you feel nervous or awkward. Follow your truest self without any expectation of you or the other person, but just practice being loving and authentic both to you and the other person.

A this point you might be thinking, "But what if they hurt me? What if they use it against me?"

Here we come back to discernment. Not everyone is ready or wants to open their heart, and that's ok. They don't know the benefits of true freedom, better support, deeper love, less confusion, more trust, and juicer, fulfilling relationships

Share your feelings with kindness and start small. You will gauge where the other person is by their response. If they continually shut you down, belittle you, or ignore any emotional conversation, this probably isn't a very healthy person to be in relationship with.

As you grow, you will want to be around people who can also be real. What I have found though, is that one if partner braves intimacy, simply stating how they feel (I feel nervous; I feel worried about; I feel very attracted to you;) it gradually opens their partner's heart and opens the door for them to be expressive and honest too.

So, intimacy starts with the bravery to tell the truth to yourself, peeking beneath the comfortable surface and getting real about how you *really* feel, not how you *think* you should feel in a given situation. Intimacy takes courage, but you can do it.

These brave conversations are the ones that address the elephant in the room, and can hear the other person's point of view without having to defend or attack. They are the conversations that express how you really feel, instead of playing games or trying to keep hold of power. When you are intimate you share power and seek to understand, rather than control.

These brave conversations help you understand your partner and yourself better, so you can have a happier relationship.

Two key questions that could save many relationships are:

What makes you feel loved?

What makes you feel unloved?

The answers will illuminate and educate you!

The trick in this process is to allow yourself and your partner to express freely. No one answer is better than another. Be sure not to let others make you feel small, just because they don't agree with your feelings.

What is your partner's 'love language?'

Some of us need kind words and 'I-love-yous,' some need undivided attention, some feel loved with a thoughtful gift, some need lots of physical affection.

Which one couldn't you live without? And what about your partner?

Be kind and clear in your communication with each other.

If you choose the Path of the Heart, love becomes a personal, spiritual practice in noticing when you choose love, and when you choose fear. Noticing which thoughts and behaviours come from your fear, and choosing instead the path of love, allows you to quickly start seeing all the beliefs you have that keep you apart from love. Your relationships become a powerful path of spiritual transformation, as you face each fear, one by one, and ask yourself if you want to carry this fear forward or release it. You commit to learning about love and healthy intimacy so you can live open-heartedly and free from fear.

This is not an easy path, but it is always worth it. The path of love is both destructive and transformative. All that is not love will spiral to the light for you to see and heal, as you root down into embodying more love and divine light in your being. Because when you release fear, love fills you up and it permeates every area of your life.

This path towards love is yours. You cannot change your partner; that is not your job. But you can fill yourself up with so much love, that people notice and want to know what it is you're doing that makes you so light and loving.

When hearts truly meet, magic happens. Intimacy doesn't require perfect, it requires authentic, whatever that is for you.

"I am not neat. Not a well-behaved woman with perfect, tidy hair and a quiet, careful voice.

I am wild and emotional and free. Overflowing with a loud love I won't contain.

I don't swim in shallow waters, for that is where alligators live."

- Jay Diamond

Exercise:

Build a vision of how you would like to be in relationships. Write a new relationship story. Who are you? How do you act and react? What kind of beliefs would you have to master to live this kind of relationship?

Summary:

* Relationships can be hard because we've never been taught how to have conscious relationships or navigate the ups-and-downs with kind and clear communication. We form a 'shell' to keep ourselves safe from hurt.

- Having the courage to be intimate, by understanding and sharing how you truly feel, will create more closeness in your relationships. Having brave conversations will transform your relationships.

- The Path of the Heart is a personal spiritual practice to help you face and let go of the fears that hold you apart from love.

Healing my Relationship with Men

Healing my relationship with men was a long, long road. As sexual abuse is often perpetrated by a family member (as in my case) or family friend, the closeness of the abuser creates a whole host of trust and intimacy issues. The mind often then creates a connection between affection, love, and familiarity with abuse.

In addition, if your parents didn't have a healthy relationship pattern, and at least one of them was abusive in any kind of way, you may find yourself replicating these same unhealthy relationship patterns or find it hard to keep a relationship going.

Although I was always clever, hardworking, and motivated, I struggled in the area of my personal relationships. I could never quite seem to get it together, and this seemed to confuse the people around me. Sure, I was feisty, but I was also loving, loyal, and although I didn't realise it, as beautiful as any other woman.

You see, the problem was on the inside.

I looked just fine on the outside, but underneath my sunshine and smiles for everyone else, I felt ugly deep down.

Not only did I experience abuse as a child, but as a teenager I was sexually assaulted again. I had terrible, greasy skin that made me self-conscious, and all the hurt in my heart made me quick to anger. As far as I was concerned, men were out to get me.

It was after a long time of deep healing work that I realised that my mind had created a link between my sexual desire and feeling used. Therefore, I didn't believe I could have both love and a good sexual relationship at the same time. And as we know, what you believe, even if it is a blind spot, is eventually what you get. I attracted a lot of emotionally unavailable men, which only reinforced my view that men were unreliable and I was not lovable.

Despite all this, I still hung on to my belief in love!

Somewhere in my heart, I desired to be in a happy, healthy relationship, even though I didn't know how to do it.

I believe everyone deserves love, no matter what you have been through or how messed up you think you are. If you commit yourself to healing your mind, body, and soul, love is available for you. There are lovers in the world looking for someone just like you because you are the perfect person for them. You have all the necessary qualities they need in a mate.

It's my understanding that we have more than one soulmate; in fact, we have many possibilities. The universe is abundant. So if it doesn't work out with one relationship, there will always be more. There is no lack of love in the universe, only our lack of seeing and believing it.

I have made many mistakes in relationships. I have been insecure, jealous, angry, fearful, and distant. But, one day I decided I would do whatever it took to overcome my fear of men. I knew logically that there were many wonderful and incredible men in the greater world, but my heart had to heal for me to see this in my own personal world.

I did three things:

I stopped what wasn't working.

I reprogrammed my mind.

I reclaimed my love for myself.

Although these precepts relate to my journey with men, the principles apply to everyone if you want to move from Abuse to Abundance in your personal relationships.

Stop what isn't working

There's so much social pressure around relationships. You're expected to marry and have kids by a certain age, and if you don't, you'll start to hear, "Your time is running out," "You'll get left on the shelf," and "What's wrong with you?"-- Especially if you are a woman.

The thing is, many of the people who said these words to me weren't in happy relationships themselves. But society expects you find someone and get involved anyway, whether or not you're happy.

I'd been through so much in my life, that I would rather be happy alone than miserable married!

I learned to be grateful where I was with what I had -- an awesome life that didn't revolve around a relationship. With no dad around, no good blueprint of how a relationship should be, and a series of disappointing relationships, I learned how to be happy and thrive on my own. This is an excellent life skill; it's just I wanted more.

In my first ever Ayahuasca journey, I deeply felt the longing of wanting to be loved.

Admitting that I really needed and wanted to be loved was so hard because I didn't believe I could have love. I felt weak and stupid that I wasn't in a happy relationship, and I had come to the conclusion that there must be something deeply wrong with me. "Love never stays," was my belief. I was so embarrassed of being a failure that I put on an, "I'm OK," outer shell for the outside world. I didn't want anybody's pity.

I wore that mask for so long, I started to believe it myself. But as the walls came tumbling down, I finally admitted, "I don't want to be alone anymore. I need someone who really cares about me."

The first step was telling the truth about what I really wanted.

The plant spirit showed me that I had allowed myself to be used by men to bolster their egos, and ego doesn't need to come into sex. I saw clearly that there were many times when I didn't feel comfortable with a man but was too afraid to speak out. There were even times that something was hurting me during sex, but I said nothing because I wanted the guy to think I was sexy and desirable.

I was more concerned about whether a man who wasn't invested in me liked me, than I was about loving myself. I had dishonoured myself.

In our society, women are conditioned to believe that our worth is about how sexually available and attractive we are for men. This idea is sold to us through magazines, television, fashion, and often through our own families. Little girls are told they're pretty; little boys are told they're clever. Mix this conditioning in with low self-esteem, and it's a lethal cocktail of self-abandonment.

By society's general standards, it doesn't matter how clever you are, or how far you get as a woman. The focus is, are you attractive?

Logically, I was so tired of that crap. Yet, the Ayahuasca showed me where I was still conditioned by it. It was still showing up in my behaviour; it was still showing up in my thoughts; it was still showing up in how I quietly compared myself to other women.

I had to take a stand and reprogram myself. Instead of trying to be attractive on the outside, I had to heal myself on the inside.

This is how you use your power as a woman, to magnetise from within, not sexualise from without.

I had come a long way from the crazy relationships that turned me upside-down and tore me inside-out. I didn't allow a man into my life any more just because he found me attractive, yet there was still a way to go. The woman in me was frozen, and I had to thaw her out.

I decided I would only connect sexually with someone if there was love. I made a commitment to myself and ended the relationship with the guy I was dating. He was nice, but it wasn't love. The uncomfortable truth was he was yet another emotionally unavailable man. I had to break the cycle.

Finally, I realised that sex really is a sacred union between two souls and should be respected as such.

Exercise:

Take responsibility for how you show up and soften your outer shell so you can build abundance in your relationships. Today is the day you can draw a line under the past and create a new, improved future.

What three things can you commit to today to improve your personal relationships?

Reprogram your mind

"The magnificence of the heart of God is your every waking moment" - San Pedro spirit

I was in a very beautiful countryside. Birds loudly sang joyful melodies, and lush green grass stretched towards the sun with pride and ease. An array of beautiful flowers offered themselves to the bees and butterflies, and the sky was baby-blue with white candy-floss clouds.

This lovely vision took place during a San Pedro ceremony; a South American plant medicine well-known to facilitate communion with nature. Harvested with great love and intention by our Peruvian shaman, the experience lasted for around eight hours and was a pivotal day in healing my relationship with men.

Relaxed and open, I sat in front of a large flower bed admiring all of the colours magnificently laid out before me. Opening my heart, I could hear the 'voices' of all the flowers in my sight. I tuned my frequency to the sounds of nature in the way shamans and healers have talked about for centuries.

Sitting beside a beautiful shrub, I laid my hands on it, feeling a pull of connection. I felt illuminated from within, and gradually the plant revealed to me my lack of compassion for men.

I was shown myself through the eyes of the men I had interacted with over the years, a reel of memories I had long forgotten. Like an outsider looking into my own life, I saw all the times my words and negative energy hurt the men in my life, whether intentionally or accidentally. Viewing myself through their eyes was a shock. I could see that I came across as cold and sometimes mean.

Because of all of my harmful experiences with men, I expected them to hurt me and it made me defensive and quick to anger. I saw threat where none was intended, and I didn't know how to communicate with men and still feel safe. I had no idea that my underlying fears and behaviour made men feel unwelcome by me.

While it's a normal occurrence to not know how to have good relationships when you've been deeply hurt, carrying the same unhealthy reactions for the rest of your life only hurts you and keeps love away.

This was the shadow side of my usually loving, generous nature; the part I didn't want to see and wasn't even aware of.

To heal my relationships with men, I had to let go of how I had learned to protect myself and build new beliefs and behaviours to love and respect men. It was the only way forward.

That didn't mean I should no longer be discerning about who I let into my life; quite the opposite. But it meant that I could learn to make choices from the present, not a dysfunctional past.

To shift my thinking, I had to form a new model of men in my mind, not one based on my earlier experiences.

I actively sought out positive male role models, and followed, noticed, and acknowledged positive masculine qualities. I stopped making men wrong, just for being men.

As I walked down the street I would say to myself, "Oh, I love how loving that man is with his children. There are so many good dads around." Or, "Wow, look at this man who is so generous with his partner. What a great guy!"

I forcibly rewired the neural networks of my brain to associate men with love and happiness, instead of fear and anger.

If you want to do this practice for yourself, get a journal and dedicate yourself to filling it up with all the positive attributes, experiences, and good things you notice on a day-to-day basis about the gender you are attracted to. Record the lovely interactions you see between couples and build new thoughts and memories of love and relationships.

If you come from a family with no examples of stable, emotionally healthy men or women, how can you be expected to know what 'normal' is or how to relate to it?

As the Wachuma plant showed me how I had seemed at times to the men in my life, I grieved the ways I unknowingly hurt men with my lack of compassion, my lack of trust, and my utter lack of relationship skills.

It takes courage to look at your own behaviours that create havoc in your life. But the truth will set you free. These unconscious behaviours are our blind spots; we build strong defence mechanisms to keep us safe, but they also keep us lonely.

I saw men through new eyes; they could get hurt, just like me. They were on their own journey in this life, one where they were expected to be strong, to suppress their emotions, and to never appear weak. I could finally see more of their humanity, their pain, and their love.

I moved from an 'Us vs Them' mentality to, *"We really are all in this together."* We're not so different deep down. I cried with relief.

These sacred plants are incredible because they are able to bypass our very solid, long-held defence mechanisms to reach **the truth in our hearts;** we all want to love and be loved. They helped me let go of the ingrained patterns of behaviour that were destroying my relationships.

As resentment left my body, light and love expanded within my body into the bliss of gratitude. I felt like a perfect, new-born baby, full of possibility and expectation. Smiling, I looked up to the bright blue sky and a cloud took the form of an Angel. She shone down on me with a divine light that filled every inch of my body with love.

"You have always been loved," she reminded me.

"It's impossible for you not to be loved!"

I immediately understood that there is indeed a constant stream of universal love flowing to us all the time; even if we can't always feel it.

It really is true that through all the good times and the bad, you have always been loved.

Many spiritual teachings tell us that love/ universe/ God is always around us, and already within us. We just have to open up and realise it. As these words became reality, my body was ecstatic. At our deepest level we are all magnificent beings.

"Your task is not to seek for love, but merely to seek and find all the barriers within yourself that you have built against it." - Rumi

Exercise:

Find your blind spots.

Ask a kind and loving friend you trust what you can work on to improve your relationships. In order to receive the support you desire, you must decide not to make your friend feel bad if they say something you don't like, as they probably will -- that's the point! Instead thank them and start working on that area of your life.

Bach flower remedies, homeopathy, and shamanic drum journeying are great places to tackle this area of reprogramming your mind, as well as using your positive stories journal. There are many experienced healers, as well as myself that can help you dive deeper in to your subconscious and assist you in releasing long-held beliefs. This is something I specialise in and really enjoy about my work.

Reclaim love for yourself

I wanted to matter to somebody. Anybody. I wanted unconditional, infallible love.

But true unconditional love? That's the stuff of God.

What I sought in people can only ever be found in a Divine higher power. Scholars and poets have written about it for generations; it's the union with the Divine I really longed for. We all have a deep pull in the belly to be fully connected and unconditionally loved, even if we suppress it at times.

And this pull? It is the universe calling us home to love.

When we cultivate the love within, love is magnetised to us. Love is your birthright. You are made up of the energy of all that is, and that is love.

Healing my relationship with men required me to love myself first and foremost, then purge old resentments, pain, and unforgiveness. Rather than talk about my own journey, I would like to share a process that will help you to reclaim love for yourself.

Ho'oponopono is an ancient Hawai'ian healing technique that I use on myself and in my workshops. Paired with mirror work, it is a powerful way to purge old pain and make room for a new self-love to emerge. Follow this technique with the prayer laid out in the accompanying workbook to refill yourself with light and high vibrational consciousness.

Give yourself time, in front of a large mirror so you can gaze directly into your own eyes.

Connecting with yourself in the mirror you will complete these four sentences:

I love you for...

I'm sorry for...

Please forgive me for...

I thank you for...

Answer these four questions seven times, each time going deeper into your heart and letting go of the past. Stay with the process as uncomfortable feelings and memories come to the surface. Let them come up and be washed away by your forgiveness and love. Forgiving yourself is one of the most important things you will ever do.

At the end of this process make a commitment to yourself.

Say your name and then, "I commit to you..."

What is the most important thing you can commit to yourself right now, after doing this process that will improve how you feel about yourself? Write this commitment down. It may be a commitment to only speak kindly to yourself. It might be a commitment to quit alcohol. It might be a commitment to only have sex with people who you are sure care about you.

Summary:

- To heal your relationships, you have to tell the truth on what isn't working for you and stop doing what isn't working.

- Reprogram your mind to see the world in a new way. Consciously seek out people and experiences that reflect the beliefs you want to have. Get a journal and record all of the great things you see that represent the people you are attracted to. What success stories can you find?

- Reclaim your love for yourself so that others can reflect that love back to you. Let go of the past and illuminate your future with healing and prayer.

MOVING INTO ABUNDANCE

You have the power to create the life of your dreams. With intention and dedication a great future is possible for you, starting now.

Refer back to this book when you need support and guidance, make sure you use the downloadable workbook at http://jaydiamond.net/abundanceworkbook/ so you can receive more healing practices to help you build an all-around abundant life.

Recovery requires commitment to yourself. There will be ups and downs, spirals and unexpected feelings, but if you keep steady in your intention to manifest an abundant life, that is what you will have.

It is my prayer that you receive healing and clarity from this book and find a way to leave the past behind and build a happier future. We are all learning how to be human, and when we realise great love is all around us and let go of fear, life opens up.

This is your time to heal. It is possible and you will do it, so keep moving forward and don't worry if you fall back in to old habits at times. Forgive yourself and move forward anyway. Visit my website www.jaydiamond.net and Facebook page www.facebook.net/msjaydiamond for articles and videos that will help you along on your journey.

Be brave in your relationships, but most of all, always be loving to yourself. Allow this wound to be your gateway into love now, as you explore the nature of life, love, and consciousness.

Make your decisions based on the confident, healthy, and incredible person you are becoming, rather than the heartbreak of the past. Now is the time to break the chains over your life and claim total freedom. You are not what others did to you. You are an incredible child of the universe who has a purpose on this Earth. Teach others what you are learning, show them how to connect to their ancestors when you have learned how, talk to them about healthy sexuality; people are crying out for mature, loving conversation from someone who cares.

Take the information in this book and run with it. Decide to love your body every day and speak kind words into your heart and those of others.

Allow yourself to receive the best that this life has to offer, because when good people do well, they do more good. Then tag me in your social media so I can see your journey, because it makes my heart explode with joy!

No more hiding, no more shame, and no more fear.

We are born to be victorious, and that we shall be.

I see the God in you,

Jay xx

Printed in Great Britain
by Amazon